ALLE ZEIT WACH
1842

Panic and Phobias

Empirical Evidence of Theoretical Models and Longterm Effects of Behavioral Treatments

Edited by I. Hand and H.-U. Wittchen

With contributions by
J. Angenendt, D. M. Clark, A. Ehlers, W. Fiegenbaum, M. Fischer, B. Garssen, E. Griez, I. Hand, M. A. van den Hout, R. King, R. Maddock, J. Margraf, W. T. Roth, P. M. Salkovskis, G. Semler, C. Wilke, H.-U. Wittchen

With 22 Figures

Springer-Verlag
Berlin Heidelberg New York Tokyo

Iver Hand, M.D.
Professor of Psychiatry
Behavior Therapy Outpatient Unit
Psychiatric University Clinic Hamburg
Federal Republic of Germany

Hans-Ulrich Wittchen, Ph.D., Dipl.-Psych.
Professor of Clinical Psychology
University of Mannheim
and Unit for Evaluation Research
at the Max-Planck-Institut für Psychiatrie München
Federal Republic of Germany

ISBN-13:978-3-642-71167-1 e-ISBN-13:978-3-642-71165-7
DOI: 10.1007/978-3-642-71165-7

Library of Congress Cataloging-in-Publication Data
Panic and phobias. Includes bibliographies and index.
1. Panic attacks. 2. Phobias. 3. Behavior therapy. I. Hand, Iver. II. Wittchen, Hans-Ulrich.
[DNLM: 1. Anxiety Disorders. 2. Fear. WM 172 P192] RC535.P35 1986 616.85′223 86-3924
ISBN-13:978-3-642-71167-1

Softcover reprint of the hardcover 1st edition 1986

2119/3321-543210

Foreword

Isaac Marks, Institute of Psychiatry, London

Human emotion seems to have changed since DSM-III burst on the world in 1980. The mere fear or anxiety that people used to feel has been transformed into dramatic panic attacks, and it has become vital to know whether 3 of these occurred over the last 3 weeks. A rash of papers has appeared proving that 'panic disorder' is a disease with a specific genetic background, childhood antecedents, biological markers, and pharmacological treatment. With alacrity 'panic disorder' has been clutched to the psychiatric bosom as proof of our medical identity.

Alas, we have been here before. Did not Benedikt in 1870 call similar symptoms 'platzschwindel', believing that the common symptom of dizziness pointed to a central disturbance in balance? Did not many later think that the usual symptom of palpitations pointed to cardiovascular disturbance at the core, leading to names like neurocirculatory asthenia, soldier's heart, and effort syndrome. Roth suggested that the symptoms of depersonalization denoted temporal lobe disturbance, and called the syndrome phobic-anxiety-depersonalization. Recently quite a few have seen hyperventilation or the fear of fear as the key. The current panic school is the latest in a long line. Successive generations pin their faith on different symptoms of a protean disorder as the root of the problem. All grasp at different parts of the elephant.

Whatever we call it, a beast of some kind does seem to be there. More parts than most were touched by the term coined by Benedikt's contemporary, Westphal, in 1871 – agoraphobia. 'Agoraphobia' is particularly apposite as some fears of various public places are prominent in most cases, and there is good reason to continue with Westphal's perceptive label. Many factor analytic studies in Europe and the USA showed that fears of public places are salient in this problem, and that such agoraphobic panic and avoidance was also frequently accompanied by other nonphobic (nonsituational) features like tonic tension and phasic panics independent of any special cue, depression and depersonalization. Unlike agoraphobia, panic is a rather nonspecific term. Spontaneous panic is almost as frequent in anxious depression as in panic disorder, while phobic panic is a hallmark of nearly all severe phobias, be they specific, social or agoraphobias.

This book is a refreshing addition to the swelling literature on anxiety disorders, much of it bringing perspective from little-known but seminal research (names and numbers in parentheses henceforth denote chapter numbers and authors). The many somatic features of anxiety leads to an overlap of panic and somatization disorders (8, King et al.). Epidemiological work in Munich (3, Wittchen) has found prevalences in the general population of agora- and specific phobias and obsessive-compulsive disorder which are remarkably close to those found in the ECA survey in the USA. Those 2 surveys, together with that of Angst in Zurich, show that such anxiety disorders are far more common than used to be thought. The female predominance remains marked among agoraphobics in community as well as clinic samples. Specific phobias are the most common phobia in the community but not in the clinic, perhaps because they are less likely to cause disability and thus urgency in seeking treatment.

A lucid critique of a purely biological formulation of panic disorder comes from

Ehlers, Margraf and colleagues (4, 6). They note that a) the familial risks for panic and generalized anxiety have not yet been shown to be independent and that there are no adoption studies to indicate whether these risks are genetic ones, and b) the strongest association of childhood separation anxiety is with adult depression rather than panics. Moreover, c) the response to lactate infusions or CO_2 inhalation by cases of panic disorder is not a specific biological marker, the higher levels of anxiety and arousal that are attained during such challenge largely being a function of their higher baseline level compared with that in controls. Similar observations were made by Maranon in 1924 about the response of volunteers to an injection of epinephrin. And the response to the cold pressor test and even just wearing a gas mask while expecting an inhalation is rather like that to lactate and CO_2.

Hyperventilation can produce some features of natural anxiety and respiration training may reduce some of these (7 – Garssen, 10 – Salkovskis & Clark). This raises several questions. What proportions of agoraphobics a) hyperventilate in response to fear, b) become frightened as a reaction to hyperventilation, c) do both in a vicious circle, d) do neither? Historically, when the agoraphobia began, in how many cases was hyperventilation a primary initiating element, a secondary complicating factor, or absent?

Two long-term followup studies from Germany (9 – Fiegenbaum, 11 – Hand et al.) add to the already impressive UK and Dutch literature showing the durability of gains in agoraphobics for 3 or more years after exposure therapy, improvement often increasing even further during followup. Mood seems to improve along with agoraphobia and social adjustment. These encouraging results suggest that exposure therapy for agoraphobia should be more widely used by mental health care providers than is often the case.

Sufferers from panic disorder with agoraphobia can now be helped much more than a couple of decades ago, though we have gone less far on the path to understanding etiology. Knowledge would advance faster if a partisan biological **or** psychological approach gave way to an integrated perspective taking both sets of factors into account, while sufferers would get a better deal from therapists who acknowledged that drugs alone are not the complete solution but have a role as an addition to exposure in some cases. The interaction between biology and psychotherapy is gradually emerging in work showing the biological consequences of habituation in animals and behavioral psychotherapy has demonstrable biological consequences which overlap with those of drugs (Marks 1986).

Marks IM (1986) Fears, Phobias and Rituals. Oxford Univ. Press, NY.

Contents

Acknowledgements

This book gives a comprehensive overview of three symposia on diagnosis, etiology and treatment of anxiety disorders, that were held at the 15th annual Meeting of the European Association of Behavior Therapy, in August 1985 in Munich. We wish to thank Johannes C. Brengelmann, Director at the Max Planck Institute for Psychiatry, chieforganizer of this meeting, for his constant encouragement in the planning and the organization of these symposia. The highly reliable cooperation of all the contributors is gratefully acknowledged as well as the help and the support of our colleagues and secretaries in the final preparation of the manuscript.

We are especially grateful to Springer Publishing House for the most efficient management of all problems and difficulties resulting from the rapid publishing process.

Contributors

Jörg Angenendt, Behavior Therapy Outpatient Unit, Psychiatrische Universitätsklinik, Martinistr. 52, 2000 Hamburg-Eppendorf, Federal Republic of Germany

David M. Clark, Department of Psychiatry, Oxford University, Warneford Hospital, Oxford OX3 7JX, Great Britain

Anke Ehlers, Department of Psychology, Philipps-Universität Marburg, Gutenbergstr. 18, 3550 Marburg, Federal Republic of Germany

Wolfgang Fiegenbaum, Department of Psychology, Philipps-Universität Marburg, Gutenbergstr. 18, 3550 Marburg, Federal Republic of Germany

Martina Fischer, Behavior Therapy Outpatient Unit, Psychiatrische Universitätsklinik, Martinistr. 52, 2000 Hamburg-Eppendorf, Federal Republic of Germany

Bert Garssen, Research Department, Psychiatric Clinic, State University of Utrecht. S vd Kolkstraat 10, 3511 HS, Utrecht, The Netherlands

Eric Griez, Department of Clinical Psychiatry, Rijksuniversiteit Limburg, P.O. Box 88, 6200 AB Maastricht, The Netherlands

Iver Hand, Behavior Therapy Outpatient Unit, Psychiatrische Universitätsklinik, Martinistr. 52, 2000 Hamburg-Eppendorf, Federal Republic of Germany

Marcel A. Van den Hout, Department of Medical Psychology, Rijksuniversiteit Limburg, P.O. Box 616, 6200 MD Maastricht, The Netherlands

Roy King, Department of Psychiatry and Behavioral Sciences, Stanford University, Stanford CA 94305/USA

Richard Maddock, Department of Psychiatry and Behavioral Sciences, Stanford University, Stanford CA 94305/USA

Jürgen Margraf, Department of Psychiatry and Behavioral Sciences, Stanford University, Stanford CA 94305/USA

Walton T. Roth, Department of Psychiatry and Behavioral Sciences, Stanford University, Stanford CA 94305/USA

Paul M. Salkovskis, Department of Psychiatry, Oxford University, Warneford Hospital, Oxford OX3 7JX, Great Britain

Gert Semler, Unit for Evaluation Research, Max-Planck-Institut für Psychiatrie, Kraepelinstr. 10, 8000 München 40, Federal Republic of Germany

Cornelia Wilke, Behavior Therapy Outpatient Unit, Psychiatrische Universitätsklinik, Martinistr. 52, 2000 Hamburg-Eppendorf, Federal Republic of Germany

Hans-Ulrich Wittchen, Clinical Psychology, Universität Mannheim, Schloß, 6800 Mannheim and Unit for Evaluation Research, Max-Planck-Institut für Psychiatrie, Kraepelinstr. 10, 8000 München 40, Federal Republic of Germany

1. Introduction

Iver Hand and Hans-Ulrich Wittchen

Since 1980, the new classification of anxiety disorders in the third revision of the Diagnostic and Statistical Manual of Mental Disorders (DSM-III) has not only stimulated research in this field, but has also provoked controversy among clinicans. In both areas, the etiological role of "panic attacks" has become the focus of attention. Panic attacks are interpreted primarily as symptoms of a biological dysfunction, having a strong genetic component. Some authors even claim a common underlying diathesis for major depression and panic disorders. This biological view has recently been extended to include agoraphobia with panic attacks, and in the forthcoming revised version of DSM-III, it may even be applied to all phobias.

From such a view, some research groups have derived the almost apodictic recommendation that biological and, in particular, pharmacological treatments are the only appropriate interventions for phobic patients. Behavioral-psychological methods are regarded as auxiliary at best.

Such a position would cast doubt not only on a wide body of basic research in the biobehavioral field, but also on numerous clinical studies that in fact demonstrate the effectiveness of behavioral-psychological methods in treating the respective anxiety disorders. A vast number of carefully controlled, clinical and experimental studies has accumulated evidence that phobias, including agoraphobia both with and without panic attacks, in the majority of patients can be treated successfully with behavioral methods, such as exposure in-vivo. For acute panic states in the context of phobic responses, several effective intervention techniques have been developed. The occurrence of panic states independent of phobic trigger situations is almost never mentioned as an obstacle to the effective treatment of phobias. Rather, problems are cited in patients with "free-floating anxiety"; in such cases specific intervention techniques had much less favorable outcomes.

After an initial state of apparent confusion and growing semantic problems, sharp controversies have developed over this biological panic concept, at least since 1983. Were panic researchers not familiar enough with the behavior therapy literature? Or were behavior therapists unfamiliar with important panic research?

In this volume, authors from different areas of anxiety research review the available literature on the background of their empirical and experimental knowledge, then to present their own research in this field. The contributors represent seven independent research centers from three European countries and the United States. The chapters of this book constitute some of the main presentations to three symposia on anxiety disorders during the 15th European Congress of Behavior Therapy. It was during the joint lunch after the final roundtable of these symposia that the idea for this volume took shape, because in spite of variations in concepts and procedures, all these authors had arrived at similar conclusions regarding the importance of there being a stronger behavioral-psychological component in the criteria for anxiety disorders in the forthcoming revision of DSM-III.

The book has three main sections: **Section I** is devoted to issues of diagnostic reliability and epidemiology. The first paper by Wittchen and Semler reports very recent findings on symptom- and diagnostic reliability of DSM-III anxiety disorders. These findings point to the need for a much stronger consensus, at least among researchers, on how to diagnose panic disorders and panic attacks. Although acceptable-to-high levels of reliability were obtained with the application of a standardized interview, very low agreement resulted from less structured clinical checklist assessments. The poor interrater reliability with the clinical checklist was due mainly to a frequent overestimation of panic attacks, probably because the interviewers neglected the strict DSM-III time and frequency criteria for the diagnosis of this disorder. In a second paper (Wittchen) data from the Epidemiological Catchment Area Program (ECA) as well as the Munich Follow-up Study (MFS) were analyzed with regard to the prevalence of panic attacks, together with or independent of other mental disorders. Results show that contrary to the assumptions of the aforementioned biological panic model and to some other recent studies, most anxiety disorders do occur without panic attacks. Moreover, no empirical evidence could be found with regard to the general applicability of the "symptom progression model", which suggests that panic attacks play a key etiological role in the development of all agoraphobias. On the other hand, results support the present DSM-III distinction of three major diagnostic groups: panic disorder and agoraphobia with and without panic attacks – the first two being clearly less frequent than the third.

Section II contains five chapters by authors from three different research groups who review current theoretical models for panic attacks and the empirical evidence for these models together with their own related research. Margraf, Ehlers, and Roth give a comprehensive review of the assumptions derived from the biologically oriented panic models of Klein, Sheehan and others. They find only weak empirical evidence for these so far. Emphasizing an interactive view of complex psychophysiological models, they suggest inadequate perception of unpleasant body sensations and faulty attribution (to danger of loss-of-control signals) as the essential pathway by which different physiological and psychological mechanisms lead to panic. This point of view is substantially elaborated in the second, related paper from this group, by Ehlers, Margraf, and Roth. Reviewing the results of attempts to induce panic attacks experimentally by lactate infusion and CO_2 inhalation, they conclude that response to these challenges cannot be regarded as a biological marker for proneness to panic attacks. Two studies conducted by this group showed that the responses of panic patients and controls were basically similar and that other stressors such as the cold pressor test, produced similar subjective and physiological effects as CO_2 inhalation. They come to the conclusion, that cognitive and learning variables are essential for more specific and treatment-relevant panic models. Similarly, but with the main focus on CO_2-induction studies, van den Hout and Griez find no convincing evidence for the view that panic is caused by underlying pathophysiological abnormalities in acid-base regulation and chemoregulatory CO_2 sensitivity.

Garssen, like Salkovskis and Clark, focuses on the hyperventilation attack as a phenomenon very similar or even identical to panic attacks. In his pilot study with agoraphobics with hyperventilation syndrome, he investigates retrospectively specific ways of cognitive processing and attribution for the development of the subjective experience of panic resulting from hyperventilation. Finally, King, Margraf, Ehlers and Maddock concentrate on somatic (cardiac and visceral) aspects of panic in their patients with panic disorder or agoraphobia with panic attacks. From the literature and from their own pilot study, they hypothesize a significant overlap of panic disorder and somatisation disorder, a significant association between phobic avoidance and somatisation (i.e. particularly high somatisation in agoraphobics), and a significant association between somatisation and social dependence. On the other hand, they postulate the independence of somatisation from a history of major depressive episodes. Further, they found that high somatisation appeared independent of both high state anxiety as well as of duration of illness. These results are discussed along with the background of related neuroanatomical and neurophysiological research.

In **section III,** three studies from three different centers on behavioral treatments for phobias with panic attacks are described in terms of their treatment rationale and their long-term outcome.

Fiegenbaum applied exposure in-vivo with "cardiac phobics". The majority of these patients were probably agoraphobics, according to the "classical" diagnostic categories in behavior therapy. Exposure in-vivo included anxiety management. The importance of "cognitive preparation" prior to exposure is emphasized, but additional "cognitive group therapy" did not add to the already profound improvements from exposure.

Salkowskis and Clark, in a pilot study, selected patients with panic related hyperventilation from different groups of phobias (including agoraphobia) for a "cognitive" treatment of their hyperventilation response. "Cognitive" treatment included the deliberate induction of hyperventilation as part of the phobic response set, which was then to be tackled cognitively. Effects of these short-term interventions generalized into all aspects of phobic behavior. The context in which this study is described is a detailed discussion of the theoretical model underlying the treatment intervention, and in this respect, as implied earlier, the paper parallels the one by Garssen in section II. Because it also investigates the psychobiological effects of stress and panic on respiration in the panic patients studied, this paper also contributes to section II.

Hand, Angenendt, Fischer, and Wilke describe a large-scale follow-up study with agoraphobics one to four years after therapist-aided or manual-aided exposure in-vivo, both modes of exposure applying two very different modes of anxiety and depression management. With multisymptomatic, repeated assessments over time, it is shown that exposure treatments are highly effective "anti-phobic/panic" as well as "anti-depressant" interventions, with some specific differences in outcome between the different modes of exposure. Particular emphasis is put on separate, detailed analyses of "gainers" and "losers" in treatment and during follow-up. In this, the study is the first to demonstrate convincingly that patients who gain from treatment also show significant-to-very significant additional gains in other "neurotic" symptomatology during follow-up.

All three studies have in common: detailed information regarding an illness-treatment model prior to the application of interventions; short treatment duration; abstinence from medication; follow-up intervals of several years and very favorable short- and long-term outcome.

The unifying element in all three studies appears to be "(cognitive-emotional) response management" – independent of the authors' labeling of their treatments as "cognitive" or "behavioral". By means of direct exposure to the previously avoided phobic situation or by laboratory procedures, all induce the main physiological-cognitive-emotional parts of the phobic response in order to then teach coping skills. Although this is not at all a new ingredient of exposure treatments, those studies that compared exposure and medication, and obtained rather negative outcomes from exposure, apparently did not use such a model.

Section I

Diagnostic Reliability and Epidemiology of DSM-III Anxiety Disorders

2. Diagnostic Reliability of Anxiety Disorders

Hans-Ulrich Wittchen and Gert Semler

1. Introduction

Prerequisite to the application of behavioral-psychological and pharmacological treatment strategies for different forms of anxiety disorders is the specification and validation of reliable diagnostic criteria. The need for reliable diagnostic criteria as well as for reliable diagnostic instruments and procedures has become even more imperative with the development of new biological treatment methods, suggested for the treatment of two subgroups of DSM-III anxiety disorders: panic disorder and agoraphobia with panic attacks. As shown by Jablensky (in press), clear diagnostic decisions, however, are not easily reached, given the fact that the classification of anxiety disorders is still controversial, and given the notorious difficulty of defining many anxiety-related symptoms.

2. Definition and Classification of Anxiety Disorders

In the literature heterogeneous groups of clinical syndromes and definitions for anxiety disorders can be found. On the one hand they refer to the great variety of so-called phobic disorders, that are primarily named and characterized by the "external triggers" of phobic (avoidance) behavior, e.g. as animal phobias, acrophobias, agoraphobias etc. On the other hand, a number of different terms were used to describe a second heterogenous group of anxiety disorders, characterized primarily by anxiety response features, such as heart or cardiac neurosis, effort syndrome, nervous exhaustion, or neurasthenia or neurocirculatory asthenia. All these terms refer to recurrent, but chronic anxiety states, characterized by symptoms like dyspnoea, palpitations, fatigue and preoccupation with somatic states. Freud (1894) introduced the term anxiety neurosis for the characterization of these disorders. This term, however, like most other terms just mentioned, has resisted all attempts to append a clearer and more reliable definition. In clinical

This research was supported in part by the Deutsche Forschungsgemeinschaft (DFG). Parts of the DIS and CIDI reliability analyses were done under a grant from the National Institute of Mental Health, Division of Biometry and Epidemiology practice, the diagnosis of anxiety neurosis subsumes three rather heterogeneous groups of patients: (a) patients with multiple phobias, (b) patients with specific somatic anxiety states and (c) patients with other neurotic illnesses with predominant anxiety and/or somatic features (Wittchen et al. 1985).

More recently, the problem of reliable classification of anxiety disorders has been addressed and approached by the Research Diagnostic Criteria (RDC), and more specifically with the third revision of the Diagnostic and Statistical Manual of Mental Disorders (DSM-III, 1980). Strongly influenced by Klein's (1967, 1978) and Sheehan's (1982) work on patients suffering from recurrent anxiety states, DSM-III has suggested the following very differentiated classification of anxiety disorders.

Table 1. DSM-III classification of anxiety disorders

Anxiety states
- Panic disorder
- Generalized anxiety disorder
- Obsessive compulsive disorder
- Posttraumatic stress disorder

Phobic disorders
- Agoraphobia (with or without panic attacks)
- Social phobia
- Simple phobia

Special emphasis is placed upon a subclassification of the anxiety states, formerly referred to as anxiety neurosis, into four groups of disorders, including obsessive-compulsive disorders. Phobic disorders have been divided into three subgroups (Table 1).

The essential features of a panic disorder are recurrent panic (anxiety) attacks, that occur at times unpredictably and are not associated with agoraphobia and are due neither to a physical nor to any other mental disorder (Table 2). The DSM-III criteria further define within the subgroup of phobic disorders a separate diagnostic group of agoraphobias (Table 3) that might or might not occur together with panic attacks. Mainly for hypothetical etiological reasons, DSM-III codes agoraphobic patients with panic attacks separately (300.21), as "agoraphobia with panic attacks".

For all these disorders careful and specific descriptions were given of all essential features constituting a diagnosis. By introducing this "quasi-operationalization" the authors of DSM-III were aiming at higher levels of reliability in the diagnostic

Table 2. DSM-III: Diagnostic criteria for panic disorder

A. At least three panic attacks within a 3 week period in circumstances other than during marked physical exertion or in a life-threatening situation. The attacks are not precipitated only by exposure to a circumscribed phobic stimulus.

B. Panic attacks are manifested by discrete periods of apprehension or fear, and at least four of the following symptoms appear during each attack:
  (1) Dyspnoea
  (2) Palpitations
  (3) Chest pain or discomfort
  (4) Choking or smothering sensations
  (5) Dizziness, vertigo, or unsteady feelings
  (6) Feelings of unreality
  (7) Paresthesias (tingling in hands or feet)
  (8) Hot and cold flashes
  (9) Sweating
  (10) Faintness
  (11) Trembling or shaking
  (12) Fear of dying, going crazy, or doing something uncontrolled during an attack

C. Not due to a physical disorder or another mental disorder, such as major depression, somatization disorder, or schizophrenia.

D. The disorder is not associated with agoraphobia

Table 3. DSM-III: Diagnostic criteria for agoraphobia

A. The individual has marked fear of and thus avoids being alone or in public places from which escape might be difficult or help not available in case of sudden incapacitation, e.g. crowds, tunnels, bridges, public transportation.

B. There is increasing constriction of normal activities until the fears or avoidance behavior dominate the individual's life.

C. Not due to a major depressive episode, obsessive compulsive disorder, paranoid personality disorder, or schizophrenia.

process. However, the few data published so far on the reliability of DSM-III anxiety disorders are rather contradictory. Although quite high interrater reliability ($\varkappa = 0.74$) was obtained in the initial DSM-III field trials for joint-ratings of different clinicians, markedly lower Kappa values of 0.43 were found for the test-retest reliability (Spitzer et al. 1979). None of the other major DSM-III diagnostic groups in that field trial had lower reliability values. Unfortunately, the authors of this paper (Spitzer et al. 1979) did not report separate reliability coefficients for each subgroup of anxiety disorders. A second group of papers dealing with the Diagnostic Interview Schedule (DIS), e.g. studies by Burke (in press), Robins et al. (1981), Wittchen (1983) were also reporting rather low reliability results for most anxiety disorders, especially for Panic disorders. These results are, however, difficult to interpret and inconclusive, because the main focus of this group of papers was the question of whether or not lay interviewers, on the basis of a fully standardized diagnostic interview (DIS) are able to diagnose DSM-III disorders the same way clinicians do.

3. Aims

It is the aim of this chapter to summarize some more recent reliability results for DSM-III anxiety disorders. Because this book focuses on panic attacks, the analyses will be restricted mainly to panic disorders and agoraphobia. In this chapter, data will be reported:

(1) on the test-retest reliability of DSM-III anxiety disorders using the Diagnostic Interview Schedule as well as its expanded, modified version, the Composite International Diagnostic Interview, that is abbreviated DIS/CIDI throughout this chapter.

(2) Furthermore, it will be examined, how diagnostic results from the DIS/CIDI compare to a more clinical approach – the DSM-III checklist by Helzer et al. (1985).

4. Methods

To examine the reliability of symptoms of anxiety as well as of diagnoses, the Diagnostic Interview Schedule (DIS, Robins et al. 1981, German version Wittchen and Rupp 1981) as well as an expanded version the Composite International Diagnostic Interview (CIDI) (German translation: Semler 1985) were used. This fully standardized diagnostic interview specifies each symptom question as well as additional "probe" questions. These probe questions are designed to evaluate whether the symptom was severe enough to cause impairment, whether the symptom was caused by alcohol, drugs or medication or whether it was always due to a physical illness or injury. Examples of some of the symptom questions for anxiety states as well as for the probe system are given in Table 4.

Furthermore, this instrument allows the use of computerized diagnostic algorithms, in order to further reduce other sources of variance in the diagnostic process. Data reported here are taken from a test-retest study using Version II of the DIS (Semler and Wittchen 1983, Wittchen et al. 1985) and a test-retest study with the DIS/CIDI (Semler et al., submitted). Although the interview was originally designed to be used by lay interviewers, we used clinicians (psychiatrists and clinical psychologists) for all interviews.

For the DIS reliability study ten inpatients with an affective or anxiety disorder as well as 52 subjects from the general population were examined. All were interviewed twice within a three-day time period with the Version II of the DIS (Wittchen 1983).

For the CIDI reliability study, 60 psychiatric inpatients of the Max Planck Institute for Psychiatry and the Bezirkskrankenhaus Kaufbeuren were also interviewed twice, using the same design as in the DIS

Table 4. "Operationalisation" of panic disorder-related questions in the CIDI (shortened and modified for this paper). In addition to codings for the presence of symptoms (NO = 1, YES = 5), the DIS/CIDI allows codings about how recent the symptom was (REC). There are six possible codes for time frames from "current" (= 1) to "lifetime" (= 6).

A. Could you tell me about one spell or attack like that?	RECORD: ______________
B. Did your spell(s) ever seem to come on for no particular reason – without anything having happened that seemed to explain them?	NO REASON ... (ASK REC) .... 5 EXPLAINED BY SITUATION .... (GO TO C) 1
REC: When was the last time you had a spell that came on for no reason?	REC: 1 2 3 4 5 6
C. Have you ever had such a bad spell that you *had* to do something about it – like telephoning someone or leaving the room or house?	NO .... (GO TO C) .... 1 YES .... (ASK REC) ... 5
REC: When was the last time you had a spell that bad?	REC: 1 2 3 4 5 6

63. During one of your worst spells of suddenly feeling frightened or anxious or uneasy, did you ever notice that you had any of the following problems? During this spell: (READ EACH SYMPTOM AND CODE "YES" OR "NO" FOR EACH. REPEAT THE PHRASE "DURING THIS SPELL" FOR EACH AND CODE IN COLUMN I).

Column I	I NO	I YES	II RECENCY					
A. Were you *short of breath* – having trouble catching your breath?	1	5	1	2	3	4	5	6
B. Did *your heart pound?*	1	5	1	2	3	4	5	6
C. Were you *dizzy* or light-headed?	1	5	1	2	3	4	5	6
D. Did your *fingers or feet tingle?*	1	5	1	2	3	4	5	6
E. Did you have *tightness or pain in your chest?*	1	5	1	2	3	4	5	6
F. Did you feel like you were *choking or smothering?*	1	5	1	2	3	4	5	6
G. Did you feel *faint?*	1	5	1	2	3	4	5	6
H. Did you *sweat?*	1	5	1	2	3	4	5	6
I. Did you *tremble* or shake?	1	5	1	2	3	4	5	6
J. Did you feel *hot or cold flashes?*	1	5	1	2	3	4	5	6
K. Did *things* around you *seem unreal?*	1	5	1	2	3	4	5	6
L. Were you *afraid* either that *you might* die or that you might *act* in a *crazy* way?	1	5	1	2	3	4	5	6

Column II
IF ANY 5 COL. I A–L *AND* Q .62 REC = 1–5, ASK FOR EACH 5 IN A–L and CODE IN COL. II:
When was the last time you (had/were SX) during an attack or spell of feeling frightened or anxious?

64. How old were you the first time you had one of these sudden spells of feeling frightened or anxious	ENTER AGE & GO TO Q. 65.
65. Have you ever had three spells like this close together – say within a three-week period?	NO .... (SKIP TO Q. 66) .... 1 YES .... (ASK REC) 5
REC: Have you had three spells in three weeks since (MO/YR)?	NO 6

study (see for more details Semler et al., submitted). Data in both studies were analyzed with the DIS diagnostic computer programs for lifetime diagnoses without using the DSM-III exclusion criteria (see for details Boyd et al. 1985).

The data reported in this paper about the CIDI versus DSM-III checklist comparison, were taken from the Munich-Kaufbeuren Collaborative Study on the comparability of different diagnostic systems (Wittchen and von Cranach 1982). The CIDI interview as well as the checklist were filled out independently by two different interviewers. Both interviews were done in a three-day time period. The DSM-III checklist by John Helzer (Helzer et al. 1985) was used as an independent clinical diagnostic interview to assess DSM-III criteria and was compared to the DSM-III diagnostic results from the Composite International Diagnostic Interview. This procedure allowed direct comparisons between the results of both methods with regard to symptoms as well as DSM-III diagnoses. All interviewers were clinicians, trained and experienced in the use of the instruments.

5. Results

5.1. Test-Retest Reliability

The test-retest reliability results – based on two fully standardized diagnostic examinations with the DIS or the CIDI – allow estimations about the "stability" of the patient's answers to specific symptom questions. The degree of agreement between both independent interviews was calculated by using three measures: the percentage agreement rate, the Kappa statistic, that adjusts the concordance for chance agreement (because Kappa is dependent on the "base rate" of the disorder, i.e. the number of "positives", the base rate is also indicated), and Yule's Y as an alternative measure to Kappa; this statistic is less sensitive to low base rates (Spitznagel and Helzer 1985).

For most anxiety disorders acceptable agreement rates with Kappa values higher than 0.5 were found in both the CIDI and the DIS studies. Generalized anxiety disorder (as assessed in the CIDI study) had markedly lower test-retest reliability scores. For panic disorders high Kappa values were found in the CIDI study, markedly lower values, however, in the DIS-study. These results can be explained by some differences in the wording of the respective items for panic attacks in the CIDI, as compared to the earlier version II of the DIS. In the CIDI, panic attacks are assessed by more specific questions, which apparently allow for a better determination of symptoms.

With regard to phobic disorders (Table 6) good Kappa values resulted only for agoraphobia – whereas low agreement scores resulted for social phobia, agoraphobia with panic attacks and for simple phobias. Kappa values for simple phobia do not indicate concordance beyond chance agreement.

5.2 Test-Retest Reliability of Symptom Questions

Table 7 summarizes reliability coefficients for all DIS/CIDI questions related to panic attacks, panic disorders and agoraphobia. Although base rates for most disorders are rather low in both studies, acceptable Kappa values were obtained for most of the questions. Symptom questions with lower Kappa values (below 0.5) in at least one of the two studies were: chest pain, dizziness, feeling of unreality, and fear of dying. As expected from the diagnostic reliability results, cited above, concordance rates for items, relevant for agoraphobia were slightly lower, as compared to the other questions.

Another important consideration in making DSM-III anxiety diagnoses is the assessment of frequencies of symptoms, as well as of time criteria. That is, the determination of age of onset of panic attacks and other phobic symptoms, as well as the determination, whether panic attacks occurred more than three times in a three-

Table 5. Test-retest reliability of DSM III anxiety disorders in the CIDI study (N=60) and the DIS-study (N=62)

DSM III-diagnosis	CIDI-study (N=60)					DIS-study (N=62)		
	Agree-ment (%)	Kappa	Yule's (Y)	N	Base rate	Agree-ment (%)	Kappa	Base rate
Phobic disorder	81	0.57**	0.66	55	21	82	0.68	40
Panic disorder	97	0.84**	0.86	59	8	64	0.47	8
Generalized anxiety disorder	72	0.41**	0.42	57	30	–	–	–
Obsessive-compulsive disorder	95	0.70**	0.81	54	7	94	0.74	7
Any anxiety disorder	80	0.58**	0.59	59	31	–	–	–

* p<0.05; ** p<0.01
– Not assessed in the DIS

Table 6. Test-retest reliability of DSM III subgroups of anxiety disorders

DSM III-diagnosis	Agreement (%)	Kappa	Yule's (Y)	N	Base rate
Agoraphobia	88	0.65**	0.75	56	16
Simple phobia	82	0.19	0.34	56	12
Social phobia	89	0.44*	0.61	55	9
Agoraphobia with panic attacks	81	0.50**	–	59	17

* p<0.05; ** p<0.01

Table 7. Test-retest reliability of anxiety-related symptoms operationalized by the diagnostic interview schedule

DSM III criteria	Study A (DIS) (N=62)			Study B (CIDI) (N=60)		
	%	Kappa	Base rate	%	Kappa	Base rate
3 Panic attacks within a 3 week period	85	0.74***	19	85	0.60**	16
Dyspnoea	78	0.55*	6	92	0.57***	9
Palpitations	100	1.00***	9	88	0.60***	14
Chest pain	78	0.53*	7	87	0.42**	12
Choking	89	0.73**	3	97	0.65**	4
Dizziness	56	0.10	6	92	0.62***	10
Feeling of unreality	78	0.55*	5	90	0.45**	9
Paresthesias	88	0.71**	3	97	0.65**	4
Hot/cold flashes	89	0.78**	5	92	0.62***	10
Sweating	88	0.71**	6	88	0.52**	12
Faintness	78	0.55*	6	97	0.65**	4
Trembling/shaking	78	0.55*	5	87	0.52***	14
Fear of dying	78	0.40	8	90	0.67***	14

* p<0.05, ** p<0.01; *** p<0.001

Table 8. Panic disorder: Comparison of DSM III checklist results (clinicians rating) with the corresponding CIDI-questions (patients self-report) (N = 192)

Panic disorder – criteria/symptoms questions	N	Agreement (%)	Kappa	Yule's (Y)	Cross-tabulation: CIDI	checklist –	checklist +
Panic attacks	192	70.3	0.22	0.26	–	115	34
					+	23	20
Dyspnoea	192	86.5	0.38	0.52	–	155	12
					+	14	11
Palpitations	192	76.0	0.26	0.33	–	130	26
					+	20	16
Dizziness	192	87.0	0.32	0.50	–	159	16
					+	9	8
Paresthesias	192	90.6	0.26	0.53	–	170	13
					+	5	4
Chest pain	192	87.5	0.36	0.52	–	159	11
					+	13	9
Choking	192	89.6	0.39	0.57	–	164	9
					+	11	8
Faintness	192	93.8	0.12	0.50	–	179	2
					+	10	1
Sweating	192	77.6	0.27	0.35	–	134	22
					+	21	15
Trembling/shaking	192	82.3	0.42	0.51	–	139	15
					+	19	19
Hot/cold flashes	192	81.8	0.26	0.37	–	147	16
					+	19	10
Feeling of unreality	192	86.5	0.21	0.42	–	161	7
					+	19	5
Fear of dying	192	82.8	0.23	0.36	–	151	14
					+	19	8
Three or more attacks in 3 weeks	192	84.9	0.40	0.52	–	149	12
					+	17	14
Phobic stimuli	192	87.0	0.39	0.54	–	156	12
					+	13	11

week period. For both groups of questions rather high concordance rates were found, when using the Intraclass Correlation Coefficient (ICC). The ICC scores for the age of onset (first occurrence) of panic attacks were 0.96 in the CIDI-study and 0.99 in the DIS- study. Lower values, however, were found for generalized anxiety (ICC=0.69) and phobias (ICC=0.78). Because of the way the ICC is calculated, these values were obtained by analysing only those pairs of interviews, where age of onset was indicated both at the time of the test- and at the time of the retest interview. If all pairs of interviews are taken into account, including those, where only one of the two interviewers indicated age of onset, the results are considerably different. For nine subjects with a probable panic disorder (15%), only one of the two interviewers coded the respective age-of-onset question in the DIS. Discrepancies were even higher for generalized anxiety disorders (N=15; 25%) and for phobias (N=17; 28%). These results, however, can not be interpreted as being indicative of severe recall problems, if timing of episodes is required. Given the predetermined symptom questions of the DIS/CIDI it is more likely that the rather high number of "severe discrepancies" indicates primarily the interviewers difficulty in deciding whether the patient fulfills the diagnostic criteria at all (Wittchen et al., in prep).

5.3 Comparison of Two Diagnostic Methods (DSM-III Checklist versus CIDI)

Another way to examine the reliability issues of DSM-III diagnoses, is the analysis of how concordant DSM-III anxiety disorders are diagnosed by two different methods. For this purpose the DSM-III checklist (Helzer et al. 1985) and the CIDI were applied by two different interviewers within a reasonably short period of time from one to four days (mean 1.56 days) to exclude the possibility of changes in the psychopathological state of the patients. As shown in Table 8 rather low concordance rates and Kappa values were found on the symptom level for panic disorders as well as for agoraphobia (Table 9). Although these results might be influenced by the low base rates of some symptoms – as indicated by the higher Yule's Y values – the cross-tabulations show a high proportion of disagreements. No clear pattern of over- or underestimation of either method could be identified. The checklist approach resulted

Table 9. Agoraphobia· Comparison of DSM III-checklist results (clinicians) with the corresponding CIDI-question (interviews)

Agoraphobia-criteria symptoms/questions	N	Agreement (%)	Kappa	Yule's (Y)	Cross-tabulation CIDI	checklist –	checklist +
Tunnels	192	95.3	0.45**	0.75		–	+
					–	179	7
					+	2	4
Crowds	192	88.0	0.46**	0.59		–	+
					–	156	12
					+	11	13
Public transportation	192	93.8	0.30	0.63		–	+
					–	177	9
					+	3	3
Outside the home alone	192	91.1	0.37*	0.58		–	+
					–	169	7
					+	10	6
Being alone	192	90.6	0.39**	0.59		–	+
					–	167	7
					+	11	7

** $p<0.01$

Table 10. Comparison of two diagnostic methods: DSM-III checklist versus CIDI

	N[1]	Agreement (%)	Kappa	Yule's (Y)	Cross-tabulation CIDI	checklist –	checklist +
Panic disorder	188	87.8	0.31*	0.49	–	158	10
					+	13	7
Agoraphobia without panic attacks	185	84.3	0.17	0.32	–	151	18
					+	11	5
Agoraphobia with panic attacks	189	91.5	0.34*	0.61	–	168	12
					+	4	5

* $p<0.05$
N[1] some interviews were excluded because of missing values

in a higher number of cases with panic attacks and symptoms such as palpitations, dizziness and paresthesias, whereas the CIDI reports more often symptoms such as fainting, feeling of unreality, and fear of dying. Also the time-related questions, whether such an attack occurred more than three times in a three week period is more often asked in the CIDI, whereas the clinician in the checklist had already decided himself, that at least one of the diagnostic criteria necessary for a diagnosis of panic disorder has not been met.

With regard to the agoraphobia criteria, the checklist approach indicated a higher proportion of patients with fear of tunnels, crowds and public transportation, whereas the CIDI more often indicated phobic stimuli such as "being alone" and "being outside the home". Generally, the analysis revealed a higher number of discrepancies than agreements between the two methods. On the diagnostic level consequently similar results were obtained. Concordance rates were not significant on the 5% level for agoraphobia (Kappa=0.17) and only slightly better for panic disorder as well as for "agoraphobia with panic attacks" (Table 10).

6. Discussion

As compared to earlier publications about the diagnostic reliability of DSM-III anxiety disorders (Spitzer et al. 1979; Burke, in press) markedly better results were found in this present analysis. For the overall test-retest reliability of anxiety disorders, a Kappa value of 0.58 was found; for panic disorders even higher values of 0.84 were obtained. This indicates that most DSM-III anxiety disorders can be diagnosed reliably if two trained clinicians apply the same diagnostic interview in a strictly uniform way. The CIDI, as well as its predecessor the DIS, can be regarded as a very useful approach to a reliable psychiatric diagnosis of panic disorders, obsessive-compulsive disorders as well as most of the phobias. But it must be acknowledged, that many clinicians probably do not like the strict symptom- and probe questions required for this diagnostic interview, only allowing very few clinical judgements. Our results also indicated that careful and specific wording for each of the anxiety-related symptoms is crucial. Whereas low Kappa values were obtained for earlier DIS studies using version II of this instrument, markedly higher Kappa values were found for the CIDI, where parts of the anxiety section were changed by the introduction of more specifically formulated symptom questions. Obviously these changes resulted in markedly higher test-retest reliability, especially for panic disorders. The lower reliability scores for agoraphobia with panic attacks seem to be mainly the result of difficulties in determining agoraphobic avoidance behavior.

In addition to the test-retest reliability issue, results indicate an urgent need for a consensus at least among researchers, how to diagnose panic disorders and panic attacks. The comparison of the standardized CIDI interview results with the more clinical checklist approach revealed a number of important discrepancies. Assuming, that all our clinical interviewers were well trained and fully complied with the interviewing rules during the diagnostic examinations, we would have to expect even more discrepancies when applying the DSM-III criteria in clinical practice and research. It is difficult to make final judgements about which of the two approaches, the DSM-III checklist or the DIS/CIDI is right or wrong. Most clinicians would probably regard the clinical diagnosis (the DSM-III checklist) as the yardstick against which to measure the performance of a standardized interview such as the DIS/CIDI.

But aside from this more political controversy, there are some empirical data strongly supporting the standardized interview approach. These data involve the problem of cooccurrence (or comorbidity) of several DSM-III disorders and the importance of DSM-III exclusion rules (see Boyd et al. 1984). DSM-III requires in the case of panic attacks that panic disorders should not be diagnosed if the disorder is due to another mental disorder, such as major depression, schizophrenia, somatisation disorder or to another physical disorder. In the CIDI, a decision involving an implicit diagnostic hierarchy is made almost exclusively at the end of the interview, after covering all diagnostic areas, whereas the more clinical approach considers these exclusions from the very beginning of the diagnostic process. This important difference obviously led to many of the observed diagnostic discrepancies between the two methods compared. The clinicians tended to diagnose more "pure" panic disorders than "agoraphobia with panic attacks" (20:9), whereas in the CIDI approach fewer "pure" panic disorders, but more agoraphobias with *and* without panic disorders were assigned. Overall the CIDI revealed 23 agoraphobias without panic attacks (compared to 16 in the checklist) and 17 with panic attacks (compared to only 9 in the checklist approach). Judging from a critical review of those patients classified differently according to both methods, we tend to favor the results of the CIDI approach. The CIDI approach guarantees that the full range of possible symptoms, syndromes and diagnoses is covered before any diagnostic decisions are made, whereas the clinical approach seems to be more likely to "overdiagnose" panic disorders.

The differentiation of anxiety states and phobic disorders in DSM-III, as well as the differentiation of patients with agoraphobia with and without panic attacks, has been strongly linked to basically biological treatment methods (Klein and Rabkin 1981). These recommendations, however, are controversial and have been opposed by behavioral-psychological researchers, who claim that exposure techniques are at least equally efficient (see chapter IV). Our results indicate that the traditional clinical approach *enhances the risk of overdiagnosing* patients with panic disorders and *underdiagnosing* other disorders, such as agoraphobia. Given that the forthcoming revision of DSM-III might give panic attacks and panic disorder an even stronger position, it will be of central importance to be more careful with the diagnostic examinations, in order to avoid wrong assignments of patients to the different treatment methods.

7. References

American Psychiatric Association, Committee on Nomenclature and Statistics (1980) Diagnostic and Statistical Manual of Mental Disorders. 3rd ed. Washington DC, American Psychiatric Association

Boyd JH, Burke JD, Gruenberg E, Holzer CE, Rae DS, George LK, Karno M, Stoltzman R, McEvoy L, Nestadt G (1984) Exclusion criteria of DSM-III: A study of cooccurrence of hierarchy-free syndromes. Arch Gen Psychiatry 41:983–989

Boyd JH, Robins LN, Holzer III CE, Von Korff M, Jordan KB, Escobar JI (1985) Making diagnoses from DIS data. In: Eaton WW, Kessler LG (eds) Epidemiologiy field methods in psychiatry. The NIMH Epidemiologic Catchment Area program. Academic Press, Orlando San Diego New York London Toronto Montreal Tokyo, pp 209–231

Burke JD Diagnostic categorization by the Diagnostic Interview Schedule (DIS): A comparison with other methods of assessment. In: Barrett J (ed) Mental disorder in the community: Progress and challenge. In press. Guilford Press, New York

Feighner JP, Robins E, Guze SB, Woodruff RA, Winokur G, Munoz R (1972) Diagnostic criteria for use in psychiatric research. Arch Gen Psychiatry 26:57–63

Freud S (1959) The justification for detaching from neurasthenia a particular syndrome: The anxiety-neurosis (1894) In: Riviere J (ed) Collected papers, Vol I. The International Psycho-Analytical Press, New York

Helzer JE, Stoltzman RK, Farmer A, Brockington IF, Plesons D, Singerman B, Works J (1985) Comparing the DIS with a DIS/DSM-III-based physician reevaluation. In: Eaton EE, Kessler LG (eds) Epidemiologic field methods in psychiatry. The NIMH Epidemiologic Catchment Area program. Academic Press, Orlando San Diego New York London Toronto Montreal Sydney Tokyo, pp 285–308

Jablensky A. Approaches to the definition and classification of anxiety and related disorders in European Psychiatry. In: Tuma AH, Maser JD (in press). Anxiety and anxiety disorders. Lawrence Erlbaum Associates Publishers, Hillsdale, New Jersey

Klein DF (1964) Delineation of two drug-responsive anxiety syndromes. Psychopharmacology 5:397–408

Klein DF (1967) Importance of psychiatric diagnosis in prediction of clinical drug effects. Arch Gen Psychiatry 16:118–126

Klein DF, Rabkin J (eds) (1981) Anxiety: New research and changing concepts. Raven Press, New York

Klein DF, Zitrin CM, Woerner M (1978) Antidepressants, anxiety, panic, and phobia. In: Lipton MA, DiMascio A, Killam KF (eds) Psychopharmacology: A generation of progress. Raven Press, New York, pp 1401–1410

Robins LN, Helzer JE, Croughan J, Ratcliff KS (1981) National Institute of Mental Health. Diagnostic Interview Schedule. Its history, characteristics and validity. Arch Gen Psychiatry 38:381–389

Semler G, Wittchen HU (1983) Das Diagnostic Interview Schedule. Erste Ergebnisse zur Reliabilität und differentiellen Validität der deutschen Fassung. In: Kommer D, Röhrle B (Hrsg) Gemeindepsychologische Perspektiven 3. Köln, pp 109–117

Semler G, Wittchen HU, Joschke K, Zaudig M, Gaiso Tv, Kaiser S, von Cranach M, Pfister H, Test-retest reliability of a standardized psychiatric interview (DIS/CIDI) – DSM-III diagnoses. Submitted

Sheehan DV (1982) Panic attacks and phobias. New Engl J Med 307:156–158

Spitzer RL, Forman JBW, Nee J (1979) DSM-III field trials: I. Initial interrater diagnostic reliability. Amer J Psychiat 136:815–817

Spitznagel EL, Helzer JE (1985) A proposed solution to the base rate problem in the kappa statistic. Arch Gen Psychiatry 42:725–728

Wittchen HU (1983) The German version of the Diagnostic Interview Schedule (DIS version 2) – reliability and results from a general population survey. Report to the Division of Biometry and Epidemiology, NIMH

Wittchen HU, Burke JD, Semler G, von Cranach M, Zandig M. Assessing psychiatric history with structured psychiatric interviews – Accuracy of recall. In prep

Wittchen HU, von Cranach M (1982) Gemeinsamkeiten und Unterschiede diagnostischer Klassifikations-Systeme – DSM-III, RDC, ICD-9, Feighner – Antrag an die Deutsche Forschungsgemeinschaft

Wittchen HU, Rupp HU (1981) Diagnostic Interview Schedule. Deutsche Version II. Max Planck Institut für Psychiatrie, München (unveröffentlichtes Manuskript)

Wittchen HU, Semler G, Zerssen Dv (1985) A comparison of two diagnostic methods. Arch Gen Psychiatry 42:677–684

3. Epidemiology of Panic Attacks and Panic Disorders

Hans-Ulrich Wittchen

1. Introduction: Contribution of Epidemiological Data to the Classification of Anxiety Disorders

Although numerous studies have been published on the prevalence rates for anxiety disorders, few such studies have used standardized psychiatric diagnostic interviews, and even fewer have used the Diagnostic and Statistical Manual of Mental Disorders in its Third Revision (DSM-III 1980). To our knowledge only the comprehensive NIMH Epidemiological Catchment Area (ECA) Program (Regier et al. 1984; Eaton and Kessler 1985) as well as a smaller epidemiological cohort study, the Munich Follow-up Study (MFS, Wittchen et al., in prep; Wittchen and von Zerssen, in press) have reported detailed prevalence rates for most DSM-III disorders by using a standardized diagnostic interview, the NIMH Diagnostic Interview Schedule (DIS; Robins et al. 1981). Neither publication, however, focusses on the analysis of anxiety disorders. Thus, with one exemption (Boyd et al. 1984) only very few epidemiological data were reported, that are relevant for the current discussions and controversies about the subclassification of anxiety disorders with their suggested different therapeutic implications (Zitrin et al. 1978).

Epidemiological data are not only prerequisite to rational estimations about the frequency of a disorder in the population as well as their biosocial "risk" factors; but such data also make possible the testing of specific diagnosis-related assumptions, made for example with regard to the onset of a disorder, the characteristics of specific syndromes, and the course and outcome of a disorder.

This research was supported by the Robert Bosch Foundation. The results are part of the Munich Follow-up Study (MFS). The MFS is a comprehensive 6–8 year follow-up investigation of former psychiatric inpatients and a general population sample. Principal investigators of the program are Prof. Dr. D. von Zerssen (Head of the Psychiatric Inpatient Department, Max Planck Institut für Psychiatrie) and Prof. Dr. H.-U. Wittchen.

To illustrate this, many authors suspect that the newly introduced DSM-III panic disorders are rather frequent, but often overlooked in clinical practice (Goldberg 1982). It is necessary therefore, to examine by means of a standardized diagnostic interview, whether the rates for panic disorder exceed the traditional epidemiological estimations by Marks and Lader (1973). In their overview of different studies prevalence rates of between 2% to 4.7% of the population in the United States, Sweden and Britain were cited. Although these figures refer to the older and much wider concept of anxiety states, they would seem to be a reasonable standard of comparison, for the combined prevalence rates of DSM-III generalized anxiety disorder and panic disorder. For phobias, extremely varying rates of between 3% (Agras et al. 1969) and 19.4% for females (Costello 1982) are cited.

A second issue of great importance is whether there is epidemiological evidence for separating panic disorder from agoraphobia and "agoraphobia with panic attacks". It has been suggested (see, for example, the overview by Goldberg 1982), that in many patients panic attacks clearly precede the occurrence of phobic avoidance behavior. Thus these authors suggest to define the panic attack as a primary "disorder", and the resulting expectant, anticipatory anxiety as secondary.

Table 1 presents a model for this assumption, suggesting possible tertiary complications, such as the development of substance abuse disorders. Given, that this model is an adequate description of the illness process for panic disorder (and perhaps for most anxiety state-like disorders, as suggested by the first draft of the revision of the DSM-III criteria, Draft DSM-III-R) this model would suggest the existence of a clear distinguishable group of patients, with an earlier onset of panic attacks. In terms of the model in Table 1 this suggests a group of patients, where panic attacks have occurred first, followed by agoraphobia and perhaps other disorders later on.

Table 1. Progression of symptomatology after occurrence of panic attacks

Occurrence of panic attacks
↓
Expectant, anticipatory anxiety ——————→ Agoraphobia
↓
Depressive symptoms, helplessness ——————→ Major depression
↓
Help-seeking behavior
Medication ——————→ Substance abuse

2. Aims

The aims of this paper are threefold:

– first a summary of "lifetime" as well as "current" (6 month) prevalence rates of DSM-III panic disorders and agoraphobia as found in the two epidemiological surveys, the MFS and the ECA will be given.

– secondly, the frequency (prevalence) of all panic disorder-related symptoms and syndromes in the community will be discussed.

– finally it will be examined, how often panic attacks precede the onset of agoraphobia in the general population and in different clinical groups. For this test the "age of onset" of the respective DIS/DSM-III-disorder, as indicated by the patient during the DIS interview, will be analysed.

3. Methods

The analysis presented in this chapter is based on two different studies: (1) The results of a survey in a random sample of the adult population. This survey is part of the Munich Follow-up Study (MFS), that examined course and outcome of treated and untreated mental disorders. (2) Data from the Epidemiological Catchment Area Program (ECA), as reported by Robins et al. (1984) for lifetime prevalence rates and by Myers et al. (1984) for 6 month rates. Both studies – the MFS as well as the ECA – used the Diagnostic Interview Schedule (DIS) by Robins et al. (1982) as a diagnostic casefinding instrument for DSM-III disorders; but they differed as to the professional background of their interviewers. Whereas in the ECA trained lay interviewers were used, the MFS interviews were carried out by clinicians (clinical psychologists and psychiatrists). Both studies were conducted in the same year, 1981, and both are based on methods of random sampling in the general population.

3.1 Description of the MFS

The Munich Follow-up Study is a comprehensive, combined 7 year follow-up investigation of 291 former psychiatric inpatients and a random general population sample of 2,037 subjects, aged 18–55 at the time of *wave 1 in 1974*. In the first wave, 1,504 (78.9%) subjects of this random sample were successfully interviewed; the rejection rate was 16.2%, and 4.9% were either never available or did not terminate the interview. Furthermore, 138 subjects with a verbal IQ lower than 85 were excluded. This left 1,366 subjects for the follow-up interviews 7 years later. The interviews at wave 1 were done by trained interviewers from a health research survey company (Infratest/Gesundheitsforschung). Interviews at wave 1 included questions to assess social, marital, and professional status; use of and attitudes toward different kinds of health services; medication intake as well as an assessment of lifestyle patterns (exercise, eating habits etc.). The primary focus of this first examination, however, was the administration of clinical selfrating scales (CSR-S, von Zerssen 1976) for the assessment of depressive and paranoid tendencies (Paranoid-Depressivitätsskala, PD-S), and somatic complaints (Beschwerdenliste, B-L); an alcoholism test-scale (Münchener Alcoholismus Test, MALT, Feuerlein 1978); and a short verbal intelligence test.

For the *wave 2* interviews in the MFS, clinicians (psychiatrists and clinical psychologists) were used, allowing a more detailed clinical examination of probable cases in the community. Because of the limited financial and personnel resources, only a part of the original sample could be selected for this more intensive, clinically oriented second wave in 1981. To ensure both, a still representative subsample of the adult general population and a high number of "probable cases", a *stratified sampling technique* was used on the basis of scores in the psychopathological rating scales (CSR-S). The following procedure was applied (see Table 2). First a 38.9% (N=532) simple random sample was drawn from the 1,366 subjects successfully interviewed in the first wave. In a second step all subjects with highly abnormal test scores in at least one of the four symptom scales (N=125), and not already drawn by the simple random sampling procedure in step 1 were added to this group of 532 subjects. This second step of adding "symptomatic high-scorers" resulted in an overall number of *657 subjects for the second wave.*

Only 501 (76.3%) of the 657 subjects in the follow-up sample could actually be interviewed in wave 2; 22 (3.3%) had died, 97 (14.8%) refused the reinterview completely, and 37 (5.6%) refused parts of it. All subjects selected for the wave 2 reexamination could be traced however. With 48% of the refusers, additional refusal interviews were conducted (see for details Wittchen and Burke, in prep.). For more details of the MFS methodology, see Wittchen and von Zerssen (in press).

3.2 Design and instruments

Data reported in this paper are based exclusively on the wave 2 interviews of the

Table 2. Selection for wave II – sampling design of the MFS

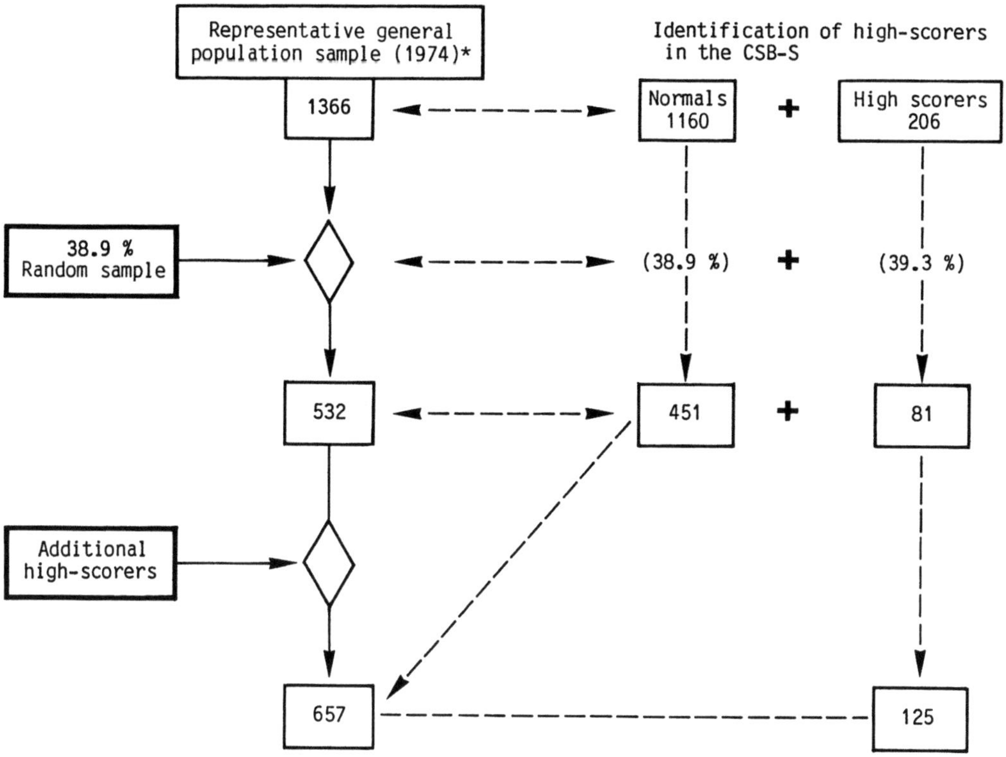

MFS. In addition to other instruments, which are described and discussed elsewhere (Wittchen and von Zerssen, in press), all subjects were interviewed with the German version of the Diagnostic Interview Schedule (Version 2) (Wittchen and Rupp 1981). The DIS is a highly structured diagnostic interview and it offers the opportunity to generate computer diagnoses according to major types of DSM-III disorders, the Research Diagnostic Criteria (RDC) and the Feighner criteria. For this report only DSM-III anxiety disorders will be considered. Generalized anxiety disorder was not included in the DIS, version II, used in this study. Although the DIS is designed for use by lay interviewers, only clinicians were used in the MFS to administer the interviews. For the test of the symptom progression model additional data from the MFS former inpatient sample were taken into account. All former inpatients with an ICD-9 diagnosis of either anxiety neurosis (300.0) or phobia (300.2) were analysed with regard to their DIS results.

3.3. Data From the Epidemiological Catchment Area Program (ECA)

All data concerning the U.S. studies were taken from the publications by Robins et al. (1984) and Myers et al. (1984). Only two of the sites of the ECA were considered, namely New Haven and St. Louis. Further, it should be noted that the age range of the U.S. study is covering all ages from young adults to old people, whereas the MFS was limited to subjects between the ages of 25 and 63. Although some data of the ECA do refer exclusively to the same age groups as those used in the MFS, only the ECA overall rates are considered here.

3.4 Analysis

Diagnoses according to DSM-III were generated by the DIS diagnostic computer program (Robins et al. 1981). The DSM-III exclusion criteria, which are optionally available in the computer program, were used only for some parts of the analysis.

4. Results

4.1 Prevalence Rates and Some Biosocial Characteristics of Agoraphobia and Panic Disorder

Anxiety disorders – as defined by DIS/DSM-III criteria – belong to the most frequent group of mental disorders in the general population. Higher rates were only found for substance abuse disorders which category includes alcohol, drug and medication abuse and dependence (Robins et al. 1984, Myers et al. 1984). Both studies (MFS and ECA) found the highest lifetime and 6 month prevalence rates for simple phobia and agoraphobia, whereas markedly lower rates were found for panic disorders, social phobias, and obsessive-compulsive disorders. Results across the different sites in the United States and the Federal Republic of Germany were generally rather similar. Due to the different age ranges in the MFS and the ECA, significantly higher rates were found in the MFS with regard to panic disorder ($p < 0.05$). If age groups between 25 and 65 alone are considered for this analysis, no significant differences will be found between the St. Louis, the New Haven and the MFS (Wittchen and Burke, in prep.). Prevalence for panic disorder is 2.4% for lifetime and 1.1% for current 6-month diagnoses in the MFS. The rates for agoraphobia are almost 2.5 times higher in all three sites compared in Table 3.

For females generally higher lifetime and 6-month prevalence rates of all DSM-III anxiety disorders were found in the MFS. Men younger than 44 had a significantly lower lifetime rate of panic disorders as compared to women of the same age range and men older than 44. On the other hand, men younger than 44 indicated a higher rate of simple phobias and obsessive-compulsive disorders as compared to older men (Table 4).

4.2 Frequencies of Symptoms and Syndromes Related to DSM III Panic Disorders

Symptoms specifically relevant for a DSM-III diagnosis of a panic disorder were found

Table 3. Lifetime- and 6 month prevalence rates of DSM-III anxiety disorders in two ECA-sites and the MFS

	DIS/DSM-III disorders prevalence rates (%)										Total	
	Panic disorder		Agora-phobia		Simple phobia		Social phobia		Obsessive compul-sive D.		Anx-iety	Dis-order
	R %	SE	R %	SE	R %	SE	R %	SE	R %	SE	R %	SE
MFS-lifetime	2.4	0.7	5.7	1.2	8.0	1.4	–	–	2.0	0.7	13.9	1.7
MFS-6-month	1.1	0.6	3.6	1.0	4.1	1.0	–	–	1.8	0.7	8.1	1.4
ECA-New Haven lifetime	1.4	0.2	3.5	0.5	6.2	0.6	–	–	2.6	0.3	10.3	0.6
ECA-New Haven 6-month	0.6	–	2.8	–	4.7	–	–	–	1.4	–	7.9	–
ECA-St. Louis lifetime	1.5	0.3	3.9	0.5	7.7	0.8	–	–	1.9	0.3	11.0	0.7
ECA-St. Louis 6-month	0.9	–	2.7	–	4.5	–	1.2	–	1.3	–	7.6	–

– not assessed

Table 4. MFS prevalence rates across age-groups and sex

	DIS/DSM-III disorders prevalence rates (%)										Total	
	Panic disorder		Agora-phobia		Simple phobia		Social phobia		Obsessive compul-sive D.		Anx-iety	Dis-order
	R %	SE	R %	SE	R %	SE	R %	SE	R %	SE	R %	SE
MFS-lifetime rates for:												
Men ≦44 age	0.9	0.7	2.7	1.2	7.5	1.9	–	–	2.5	0.9	10.1	2.2
Men >44 age	3.6	1.2	3.0	1.4	3.2	1.2	–	–	1.0	0.8	7.9	2.0
Men total	1.7	0.7	2.9	0.9	5.5	1.1	–	–	1.8	0.6	9.1	1.5
Female ≦44 age	2.8	0.9	8.5	1.9	10.9	2.1	–	–	1.3	0.8	16.4	2.5
Female >44 age	3.0	1.3	7.9	2.1	9.5	2.3	–	–	3.4	1.3	19.8	3.1
Female total	2.9	0.8	8.3	1.4	10.4	1.6	–	–	2.3	0.8	18.1	2.0

– not assessed

Table 5. MFS frequency of panic disorder-related symptoms in the general population (prevalence rates)

DIS/DSM-III symptoms	Males			Females			Total
	Total R %	≦44 R %	>44 R %	Total R %	≦44 R %	>4 R %	R %
Panic attacks	7.1	5.9	8.5	11.1	11.6	10.3	9.3
Dyspnoea	3.9	1.8	6.3	7.1	7.0	7.0	5.6
Palpitations	7.4	5.9	9.1	11.4	12.5	9.8	9.6
Dizziness	4.2	0.9	8.1	3.8	3.9	3.8	4.1
Paresthesias	2.0	–	4.2	3.3	5.4	0.9	2.6
Chest pain	4.8	4.1	5.7	6.4	5.7	7.0	5.7
Choking	3.6	2.7	4.7	3.1	2.2	4.0	3.5
Faintness	2.9	4.1	1.6	4.3	4.1	4.5	3.7
Sweating	6.1	6.8	5.4	7.7	9.2	5.8	7.1
Trembling/shaking	3.2	1.8	4.8	8.0	9.1	6.7	5.7
Hot/cold flashes	5.7	5.0	6.5	6.9	8.1	5.4	6.3
Feeling of unreality	3.2	–	6.9	4.1	5.9	1.9	3.7
Fear of dying	3.9	2.7	5.3	7.0	8.1	5.7	5.6
3× in 3 weeks	3.7	1.8	5.9	4.8	4.4	5.0	4.3

to be rather common in the general population, when a standardized diagnostic procedure, such as the DIS is used. The overall rate for panic attacks, as assessed with the DIS was 9.3% (Table 5); and thus was almost three times higher than the combined prevalence rates for panic disorder and "agoraphobia with panic attacks". With a few exceptions (symptoms of choking, dizziness) females indicated more often specific somatic symptoms, that occurred together with a panic attack, 11.1% of adult females (aged 25–63 at the time of examination) and 7.1% of all males reported having had, at least once in their life, a panic attack. For almost two-thirds of them, this attack was accompanied by at least four of the 12 symptoms, necessary for a DSM-III diagnosis of panic disorder.

On the other hand, only 3.7% of all male and 4.8% of all female patients had had such an attack "more than three times in a

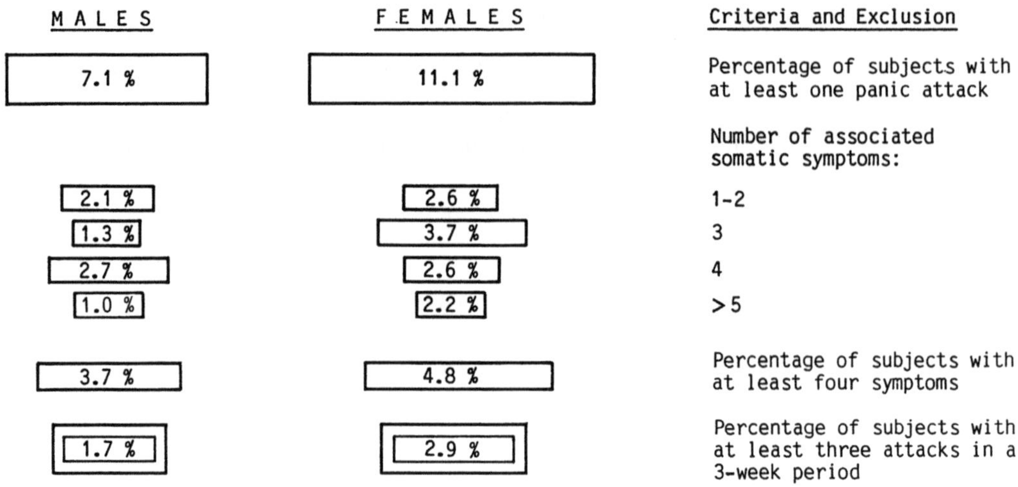

Fig. 1. "Hierarchy" of panic disorder-related symptoms and syndromes in male and female patients and the observed frequency in the population

Table 6. MFS – General population sample: anxiety disorders (panic, phobic disorders only) and their age of onset

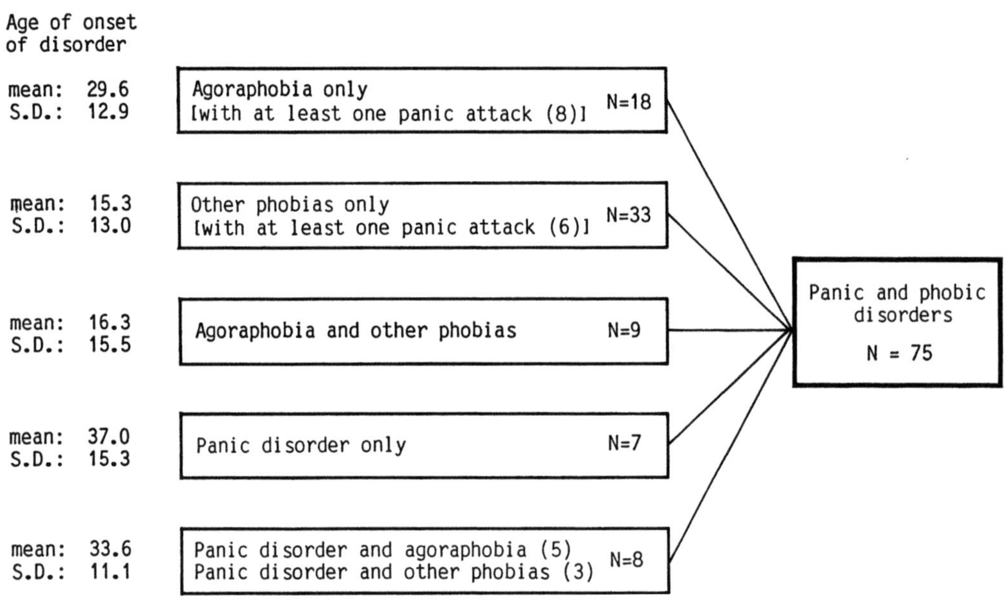

3-week-period", as defined by the DSM-III criteria. When the exclusion rules for panic disorder are taken into account, the results are a 1.7% rate for males and a 2.9% rate for females.

The hierarchy of DSM-III diagnostic decisions (Fig. 1) clarifies, that only a small percentage of subjects who have ever experienced panic attacks actually obtain the diagnosis of a panic disorder. Most do not fulfill either the criteria for the necessary number of somatic symptoms or the time, frequency, and exclusion criteria.

4.3 Age of Onset of Anxiety Disorders

The DIS allows the determination of the age of onset for most diagnostic sections by asking for the first occurrence of the disorder, whose primary diagnostic criteria have been met. The following data refer to these age-of-onset questions, which are asked separately for panic disorder and phobias (see for examples of these DIS-questions the chapter by Wittchen and Semler). The analysis in Table 7 takes into account the MFS-general population survey data, as well as the Munich-Follow-up Study former-inpatient-sample data of those patients with an ICD-9 anxiety disorder of anxiety neurosis (ICD-9 No. 300.0) or phobia (ICD-9 No. 300.2). The temporal cooccurrence of panic attacks and phobic avoidance behavior found in more than half of both samples was counted as positive in this analysis with regard to the hypothesis that panic attacks precede agoraphobia.

In the MFS general population survey (Table 6), 75 subjects received a lifetime DSM-III diagnosis of either panic disorder and/or any other phobic disorder. Table 6 shows the resulting diagnostic subclassification for these 75 "cases", not taking into account DSM-III exclusion rules. Of the 75 "cases" 18 received a lifetime diagnosis of agoraphobia, 33 of some other DSM-III phobic disorder, nine cases had both, agoraphobia as well as some other phobia. Only a small proportion (N = 15, 20%) of the overall group fulfilled the DSM-III diagnostic criteria for panic disorder: seven of them without any phobic avoidance behavior, five with agoraphobia and another three patients with other phobias.

It must be noted, that a remarkably high number of cases who met diagnostic criteria of phobic disorders (simple phobia, social phobia, agoraphobia) also indicated at least one, but not more than three panic attacks in a 3 week period. Thus, eight of the 18 agoraphobics and six of the 33 "cases" with phobic disorders (as indicated in the brackets in Table 6), had panic attacks below the diagnostic threshold. The age of onset, that is, the year of the first occurrence of a specific DSM-III anxiety disorder, showed a lot of variation among subjects. Generally cases with phobic disorders, especially simple and social phobias (mean age: 15.3 years) revealed a lower age of onset of their disorder than cases with agoraphobia (mean age: 29.6) or panic disorders (mean age: 37.0).

An analysis of cases and patients, who fulfilled the criteria for both, panic disorder and phobic disorder, revealed that in the majority of cases the first occurrence of

Table 7. Phobic disorders with panic disorder or at least one panic attack. Time sequence (age of onset)

	MFS-general population – anxiety cases –					Former inpatients with ICD-9 anxiety disorders (300.2/300.0)				
	Yes		No		Total	Yes		No		Total
	N	%	N	%	(N)	N	%	N	%	(N)
Model 1: Panic disorder ⟶ Agoraphobia ⟶ t	4	80	1	20	5	13	93	1	7	14
Model 2: Panic disorder ⟶ Any phobias ⟶ t	5	63	3	27	8	15	94	1	6	16
Model 3: Panic attacks ⟶ Agoraphobia ⟶ t	11	73	4	27	15	12	75	4	25	16

t = time axis

panic attacks either preceded or accompanied the first manifestation of phobic avoidance behavior (see Table 7). This relationship could also be ascertained for those 15 cases and 16 former inpatients who only indicated an occurrence of panic attacks below the DSM-III diagnostic threshold.

5. Discussion

Anxiety disorders, as defined by the DIS/DSM-III criteria belong to the most common mental disorders in the community. The lifetime prevalence rates in all three studies compared in this paper (Robins et al. 1984; Myers et al. 1984; Wittchen et al., in prep.) varied between 10.3% and 13.9%, the 6-month rates between 7.6% and 8.1%. In interpreting these results, however, it should be noted that generalized anxiety disorder was not included in these estimations. Therefore the "true" overall rates for anxiety disorders might even be slightly higher.

Compared with the overall prevalence of anxiety disorders, panic disorders are rather rare. The 6-month prevalence rates were 0.6% in the New Haven site of the ECA (Meyers et al. 1984) and 1.1% in the Munich Follow-up Study (Wittchen and Burke, in prep.). The lifetime rates were slightly higher, ranging between 1.4% and 2.4%. This finding is in accordance with earlier studies by Weissman et al. (1984) using the SADS-L version to assess the Research Diagnostic Criteria for panic disorder. They reported a 6-month prevalence rate of 0.4% for the last 6-month period before the interview. Agoraphobia was found to be generally more frequent in all three sites. Lifetime rates varied between 5.7% and 3.7%. Because these DIS/DSM-III prevalence data were analysed without using the exclusion rules for other mental disorders, there is some overlap of panic disorders and agoraphobia. By taking into account the exclusion rules, one third of the cases with panic disorders were classified as agoraphobia with panic attacks.

Altogether these results suggest that neither panic disorder nor agoraphobia with panic attacks are more common than suggested by earlier estimations by Lader and Marks (1973), if a standardized diagnostic procedure is used.

It is also important to note that many symptoms, specified for the diagnosis of panic disorder are very common in the population. The overall rate for panic attack-like symptoms, as assessed with the DIS, was 9.3% and thus was almost three times higher than the combined prevalence rates for agoraphobia with panic attacks and panic disorders. The high prevalence rates for panic disorder-like symptoms underscores the need for a very careful diagnostic evaluation to assess the criteria for both panic disorder and panic attacks in agoraphobia. As shown in the hierarchy of criteria, special attention must be paid in this context to the assessment of time, and frequency- and exclusion-criteria.

Concerning gender differences, it was found that women are affected by panic disorders almost twice as often as men. Although this result has already been mentioned in a number of previous studies, most of these have been biased by the use of exclusively clinical samples. The preponderance of females was found to be even more pronounced in agoraphobia, with rates almost three times higher for women than for men.

With regard to the age of onset of panic and phobic disorders, clear differences were found. Generally, simple phobias as well as social phobias had an earlier onset, whereas agoraphobias and panic disorders occurred significantly later in a given patient's life. On the basis of the age-of-onset data the "symptom progression model" suggested by Goldberg (1982) was partly confirmed. In most subjects with at least one panic attack and agoraphobia, panic attacks as well as panic disorder did either precede or occur together with agoraphobic avoidance behavior. But it must also be noted that many (almost 50%) of the cases/patients with agoraphobia had never experienced either a panic attack-like state, or the full picture of a panic disorder. Although the limitations of the present study (low number of patients, retrospective assessment, no reference to data from genetic and family studies, small coverage of possible risk factors) have to be taken into account, our result underlines the importance of retaining agoraphobia as a distinct diagnostic category and supports the present DSM-III classification approach in which panic disorder, agoraphobia with and without panic attacks are defined. For panic disorder as well as for agoraphobia with panic attacks the "symptom progression model" can be regarded as a helpful prognostic model in further research.

6. References

Agras WS, Sylvester D, Oliveau D (1969) The epidemiology of common fears and phobias. Compreh. Psychiatry 10:151–156

Boyd JH, Burke JD, Gruenberg E, Holzer CE, Rae DS, George LK, Karno M, Stoltzman R, McEvoy L, Nestadt G (1984) Exclusion criteria of DSM-III: A study of cooccurrence of hierarchy-free syndromes. Arch Gen Psychiatry 41:983–989

Cloninger CR, Martin RL, Clayton PJ, Guze SB (1981) A blind follow-up and family study of anxiety neurosis: Preliminary analysis of the St. Louis 500. In: Klein DF, Rabkin JD (eds) Anxiety: New research and changing concepts. Raven Press, New York

Cohen ME, Badal DW, Kilpatrick A, Reed EW, White PD (1951) The high familial prevalence of neurocirculatory asthenia (anxiety neurosis, effort syndrome). Amer J Genetics 3:126–158

Costello CG (1982) Fears and phobias in women: A community study. J Abn Psychol 91:280–286

Crowe RR (1985) The genetics of panic disorder and agor. Psychiat Dev 2:171–186

Crowe RR, Noyes R, Pauls DL, Slyman D (1983) A family study of panic disorder. Arch Gen Psychiatry 40:1065–1069

Eaton WW, Kessler LG (eds) (1985) Epidemiologic field methods in psychiatry. The NIMH Epidemiologic Catchment Area program. Academic Press, Orlando San Diego New York London Toronto Sydney Tokyo

Feuerlein W, Küfner H, Ringer C, Antons K (1979) – MALT – Münchner Alkoholismustest-Manual. Beltz, Weinheim

Goldberg RJ (1982) Anxiety: A guide to biobehavioral diagnosis and therapy for physicians and mental health clinicians. Medical Examination Publishing Co., Inc., New York

Klein DF (1981) Anxiety reconceptualized. In: Klein DF, Rabkin J (eds) Anxiety: New research and changing concepts. Raven Press, New York, pp 235–263

Marks IM, Lader M (1973) Anxiety states (anxiety neurosis): a review. J Nerv Ment Dis 156:3–18

Myers JK, Weissman MM, Tischler GL, Holzer CE, Leaf PJ, Orvaschel H, Anthony JC, Boyd JH, Burke JD, Kramer M, Stoltzman R (1984) Six month prevalence of psychiatric disorders in three communities: 1980–1982. Arch Gen Psychiatry 41:959–967

Noyes R, Clancy J, Crowe RR, Slyman D (1978) The familial prevalence of anxiety neurosis. Arch Gen Psychiatry 35:1057–1059

Regier DA, Myers JK, Kramer M, Robins LN, Blazer DG, Hough RL, Eaton WW, Locke BZ (1984) The NIMH Epidemiological Catchment Area program. Historical context, major objectives and study population characteristics. Arch Gen Psychiatry 41:934–941

Robins LN, Helzer JE, Croughan J, Ratcliff KS (1981) National Institute of Mental Health. Diagnostic Interview Schedule. Its history, characteristics and validity. Arch Gen Psychiatry 38:381–389

Robins LN, Helzer JE, Orvaschel H, Anthony JC, Blazer DG, Burnam A, Burke JD jr (1985) The Diagnostic Interview Schedule. In: Eaton WW, Kessler LG (eds) Epidemiologic field methods in psychiatry. The NIMH Epidemiologic Catchment Area program. Academic Press, Orlando San Diego New York London Toronto Montreal Sydney Tokyo, pp 143–170

Robins LN, Helzer JE, Ratcliff KS, Seyfried W (1982) Validity of the Diagnostic Interview Schedule, version II: DSM-III diagnoses. Psychol Med 12:855–870

Robins LN, Helzer JE, Weissman MM, Orvaschel H, Gruenberg E, Burke JD, Regier DA (1984) Lifetime prevalence of specific psychiatric disorders in three sites. Arch Gen Psychiatry 41:949–958

Spitzer RL, Endicott J, Robins E (1978) Research Diagnostic Criteria: Rationale and reliability. Arch Gen Psychiatry 35:773–782

Weissman MM, Myers JK, Harding P (1978) Psychiatric disorders in a United States urban community: 1975–1976. Amer J Psychiat 135:459–462

Wittchen HU, Rupp HU (1981) Diagnostic Interview Schedule. Deutsche Version II. Max

Planck Institut für Psychiatrie, München (unveröffentlichtes Manuskript)
Wittchen HU, von Zerssen D (1986) Verläufe behandelter und unbehandelter Depressionen und Angststörungen. Klinisch-psychiatrische und epidemiologische Aspekte der Münchener 7-Jahres Follow-up Studie (MFS) (In press). Springer, Berlin Heidelberg New York
Wittchen HU, Burke JD DIS/DSM-III prevalence rates of mental disorders in the US and Germany. In prep
Zerssen Dv, unter Mitarbeit von Koeller DM (1976) Klinische Selbstbeurteilungsskalen (KSb-S) aus dem Münchner Psychiatrischen Informationssystem (PSYCHIS München). Manuale a) allgemeiner Teil b) Paranoid-Depressivitätsskala c) Befindlichkeitsskala d) Beschwerdenliste. Beltz, Weinheim
Zitrin CM, Klein DF, Woerner MG (1978) Behavior therapy, supportive psychotherapy, imipramine and phobias. Arch Gen Psychiatry 35:307–316

Section II

Theoretical Models and Empirical Evidence

4. Panic Attacks: Theoretical Models and Empirical Evidence

Jürgen Margraf, Anke Ehlers, and Walton T. Roth

1. Introduction

Panic attacks are states of intense anxiety with an abrupt onset. They are accompanied by predominantly somatic symptoms like palpitations, dyspnea, and paresthesias. In spite of Freud's (1895a) early description of panic attacks ('Angstanfälle'), psychiatry and psychology did not attach any special relevance to this form of anxiety until recently. With the introduction of the third edition of the Diagnostic and Statistical Manual of Mental Disorders of the American Psychiatric Association (DSM-III, APA 1980), official psychiatric classification acknowledged panic attacks as important features in anxiety disorders. The next revision of DSM (DSM-III-R) will emphasize even more the role of panic attacks in the classification and etiology of anxiety disorders (Spitzer and Williams 1984, Spitzer 1985).

The renewed interest in panic attacks was initiated by Klein's work on panic attacks and agoraphobia (Klein 1981). The observation that patients suffering from recurrent attack-like anxiety benefited from tricyclic antidepressants (Klein and Fink 1962; Klein 1964; Mendel and Klein 1969), led Klein to postulate a qualitative distinction between spontaneous panic attacks and other types of anxiety. He regards panic attacks as a biological dysfunction with a

Preparation of this manuscript was supported in part by the Medical Research Service of the Veterans Administration. A portion of this material was presented at the Annual Meeting of the West Coast College of Biological Psychiatry, Palo Alto, April 1985, and at the 15th Annual Meeting of the European Association for Behaviour Therapy, Munich, August 1985.

strong genetic component, a viewpoint currently shared by many psychiatric researchers on anxiety. Klein and other authors favoring *biological* models of panic, consider psychotherapy, including behavioral approaches, irrelevant to the treatment of panic attacks and recommend pharmacological treatment (Klein 1981; Shader et al. 1982; Sheehan 1982).

Other authors have approached panic attacks from a completely different perspective that has been called the *cognitive* (Clark et al. 1985) or *psychophysiological* model (Margraf et al. 1986). This approach does not assume a basic distinction between panic and other forms of anxiety. Panic attacks are explained by an interaction of physiological changes and psychological reactions. Psychological interventions for panic attacks based on these models have been devised (Goldstein 1982; Barlow et al. 1984; Bonn et al. 1984; Clark et al. 1985).

In this chapter, we shall discuss biological and psychophysiological models of panic attacks in terms of their respective status of empirical support. Other aspects of the etiology of agoraphobia and panic disorder have recently been reviewed by Roth (1984) and Foa et al. (1984).

2. Biological Models of Panic Attacks

2.1. Klein's and Sheehan's Models

Klein's model of agoraphobia and panic attacks (Klein 1981) makes a *qualitative* distinction between what he terms 'panic' anxiety and 'anticipatory' anxiety. *Panic* anxiety consists of attack-like occurrences of a group of predominantly somatic symptoms and is considered to represent a specific biological dysfunction. The attacks often occur spontaneously. *Anticipatory* anxiety on the other hand is triggered by specific stimuli and has a more chronic course. This form of anxiety has fewer and slower fluctuations and predominantly cognitive symptoms. Thus Klein's notion of anticipatory anxiety includes situational as well as tonically elevated anxiety. In the agoraphobia syndrome, anticipatory anxiety is seen as a typical consequence of spontaneous panic attacks. The patient fears the recurrence of panic and starts to avoid situations in which an attack is likely to occur. The same sequence was already conceptualized by Freud 90 years ago (1895 b).

In Klein's model, separation anxiety is related to panic attacks because both involve an unlearned alarm mechanism that is activated by separation from attachment stimuli. This innate mechanism consists of protest and despair components similar to Bowlby's first two stages of the response to separation (Bowlby 1969, 1973). The protest component includes active, help-seeking behavior (parallel to panic); the despair component includes passive behavior (parallel to depression). Klein assumes that in panic patients the threshold for this alarm mechanism is chronically lowered by some biological dysfunction. This leads to its activation by minimal triggers or even without triggers.

In a similar way, Sheehan (1982; Sheehan and Sheehan 1983) postulates "spontaneous panic attacks" as an entity distinct from other anxiety states. He proposes to classify anxiety disorders according to the presence or absence of these attacks. Phobias occurring in the presence of panic attacks are classified as "endogenous phobic anxiety" (in contrast to "exogenous"). Sheehan claims that panic attacks represent a "metabolic disease" (Sheehan and Sheehan 1983; Carr and Sheehan 1984). Secondary to this metabolic core disease and superimposed on it, learning processes can lead to the phobic avoidance behavior that is manifest in agoraphobia (see Sheehan and Sheehan (1983) for a description of the natural history of panic disorder). Even though an influence of stressors is acknowledged, they are considered non-specific exacerbating rather than causal factors.

According to Klein and Sheehan, a pharmacological treatment of panic attacks is necessary to treat panic disorder and agoraphobia with panic attacks. The treatment of situational or tonically elevated anxiety alone (e.g. by behavior therapy or diazepam) should not result in lasting improvement, since spontaneously recurring attacks would make a relapse very probable.

In the following section, we will discuss the five major arguments put forward by Klein for the validity of his model. With the exception of the analogies with separation anxiety, these arguments are also used by Sheehan.

2.2. Empirical Evidence

2.2.1. Specificity of Drug Treatment

It is argued that different drugs are therapeutic for panic and 'anticipatory' (situational or tonically elevated) anxiety. First, tricyclic antidepressants and MAO inhibitors specifically treat panic but not anticipatory anxiety. Second, sedatives and minor tranquilizers, especially benzodiazepines, do not affect panic but treat anticipatory anxiety.

This argument is not supported by the majority of drug therapy studies. First, the differential efficacy of tricyclic antidepressants is largely untested. There are as yet no published studies on the effects of antidepressants in patients with a chief complaint of generalized anxiety. However, in several studies of patients with other primary diagnoses, tricyclic antidepressants significantly reduced generalized anxiety (cf. Mathews et al. 1981; Marks 1983). Klein (1984) cites a study in press (Kahn et al., in press) in which tricyclics apparently reduced anxiety in anxious patients without panic attacks. Reviewing the topic, Marks (1983) concludes that tricyclics have a broad spectrum of effects not limited to dysphoria or panic attacks.

The second part of the drug specificity argument is challenged by the efficacy of alprazolam, a new benzodiazepine, in the treatment of both anticipatory and panic anxiety (Chouinard et al. 1982; Shader et al. 1982; Sheehan 1982). This cannot simply be a consequence of the special chemical structure of alprazolam since even the standard benzodiazepine, diazepam, recently has been shown to reduce the frequency of panic attacks (Noyes et al. 1984). This double-blind comparison of diazepam, propanolol, and placebo is the only study in which high doses of diazepam were administered to panic attack patients at regular intervals.

In addition to these limitations in drug specificity, there are several problems concerning the use of antidepressants (tricyclics and MAO inhibitors) in panic attack patients. The mechanism of their action remains unclear. Other hypothetical mechanisms besides Klein's postulation of a direct blockade of panic attacks by an (as yet unknown) biological mechanism have been suggested (Marks 1983: depression-mediation mechanism; Telch et al. 1985: exposure-facilitation mechanism). In addition, beneficial effects of these drugs have so far only been established in relatively short-term studies. Their long-term outcome is unknown (Grunhaus et al. 1981; Matuzas and Glass 1983; Telch et al. 1983; Klein 1984) and relapse rates after discontinuation may be high (Pohl et al. 1982; Keefe and Agras 1983; Marks 1983).

2.2.2. Panic Induction

It is argued that panic attacks can be experimentally induced by specific biological agents (sodium lactate infusion and carbon dioxide inhalation) in panic patients but not in normal controls. A specific biological vulnerability of panic patients is inferred.

The empirical support for this argument is far from unequivocal. A detailed review of this argument can be found in the chapter by Ehlers, Margraf, and Roth in this book. The results of this review and our own data are not compatible with the interpretation of the response to lactate or carbon dioxide (CO_2) as a biological marker for panic attacks.

2.2.3. Family and Twin Studies

It is claimed that family and twin studies show a strong genetic factor for panic that is independent from the risk for situational or tonically elevated ('anticipatory') anxiety.

One problem in evaluating the status of empirical support for this argument is that only the most recent family and twin studies are based on DSM-III diagnoses and report data on panic disorder (Raskin et al. 1982; Crowe et al. 1983; Leckman et al. 1983; Torgersen 1983). In addition, there are several family studies of agoraphobia (Solyom et al. 1974; Buglass et al. 1977; Burns and Thorpe 1977; Harris et al. 1983; Moran and Andrews 1985). Most of the studies, however, were conducted before the introduction of DSM-III (McInnes 1937; Brown 1942; Wheeler et al. 1948; Cohen et al. 1951; Slater and Shields 1969; Noyes et al. 1978; Carey and Gottesman 1981; Cloninger et al. 1981).

Most studies found an increased familial risk for anxiety disorders as well as higher concordance rates for monozygotic than dizygotic twins. However, the data on agoraphobia in particular are contradictory (Solyom et al. 1974; Buglass et al. 1977; Burns and Thorpe 1977; Harris et al. 1983; Moran and Andrews 1985). It also remains unresolved whether generalized anxiety is familially transmitted (Slater and Shields 1969; Carey and Gottesman 1981; Crowe et al. 1983; Leckman et al. 1983; Torgersen 1983). Furthermore, most studies that investigated gender effects found a significantly increased risk for anxiety disorders only or mainly in female relatives (Solyom et al. 1974; Burns and Thorpe 1977; Cloninger et al. 1981; Crowe et al. 1983; Harris et al. 1983; Moran and Andrews 1985).

While the claim of a genetic factor for panic independent of generalized ('anticipatory') anxiety seems to be supported by Torgersen (1983), Raskin et al. (1982) did not find differential incidences of panic and generalized anxiety in families of patients with one or the other disorder. Similarly, the data of Leckman et al. (1983) from depressed and anxious patients also do not show an independent familial transmission of panic and generalized anxiety.

Thus, we cannot yet say whether familial risks for panic and generalized anxiety are independent. Nor are there any adoption studies which alone would enable us to determine whether these risks are genetic ones.

2.2.4. Spontaneity of Panic Attacks

It is claimed that the majority of panic attacks especially at the onset of the disorder occur spontaneously, that is, not in response to specific stimuli.

This argument is based entirely on clinical impressions. Neither Klein nor Sheehan quote any systematic studies. Moreover, a number of recent studies point in an opposite direction. First, there is substantial evidence that nonspecific psychological or physiological stressors are related to the overall frequency of panic attacks (Brehony and Geller 1981; Mathews et al. 1981; Raskin et al. 1982; Tearnan et al. 1984; Uhde et al. 1985). Klein (1964) himself originally reported a relationship between the onset of panic disorder and "endocrine fluctuations" such as those associated with child birth or menopause in a subgroup of patients. Furthermore, precipitating events operating in a time frame of days or hours can be important for the occurrence of panic attacks (Brehony and Geller 1981; Mathews et al. 1981; Raskin et al. 1982). In addition, a study by Finlay-Jones and Brown (1981) suggests a degree of specificity of life events related to panic disorder. They found a greater frequency of "danger"-related events preceding the onset of anxiety and panic symptoms. "Loss"-related events on the other hand were more closely related to depression.

Second, most central to the validity of current biological models of panic attacks is whether immediate triggers for individual panic attacks can be found. If external or internal triggers are regularly present, the distinction between panic and other kinds of anxiety is blurred. As we will discuss in our presentation of the psychophysiological models, investigations using more systematic methods than simple clinical interviews suggest triggers for at least some individual panic attacks. Especially internal cues are promising candidates for such triggering events. These include bodily sensations that are interpreted as dangerous and anxiety-inducing thoughts and images.

2.2.5. Separation Anxiety and School Phobia

Klein argues that separation anxiety in young animals and 'school phobia' in children responds to treatment with tricyclic antidepressants. Second, he claims that about half of all agoraphobic patients have a childhood history of separation anxiety.

In animal studies, positive effects of imipramine on distressed behavior following separation were observed (Scott et al. 1973; Suomi et al. 1978). The success of tricyclic antidepressants in treating 'school phobia', however, is not yet well established. While Gittelman-Klein and Klein (1973, 1980) reported a positive effect of imipramine in doses of up to 200 mg, Berney et al. (1981) found no effect of a lower dose of up to 75 mg of clomipramine. Furthermore, a history of separation anxiety does not correlate with therapeutic success of imipramine in the treatment of agoraphobia (Gittelman-Klein and Klein 1984). In addition, there is no evidence for a genetic transmission of a vulnerability for separation anxiety from agoraphobic parents to their children (Berg 1976; Gittelman-Klein 1975).

Klein and his coworkers have conducted several studies that show an elevated incidence of childhood and current separation anxiety in panic attack patients (Klein 1964; Gittelman-Klein and Klein 1984). In a series of better standardized and controlled studies by other groups, no differences were found between agoraphobic or panic disorder patients and control subjects or other anxiety patients in difficulties in attending school ('school phobia'), signs of separation anxiety, the death of a parent, or the frequency of permanent or longer-term childhood separation from the parents (Berg et al. 1974; Solyom et al. 1974; Buglass et al. 1977; Raskin et al. 1982). Reviewing the etiology of agoraphobia, Tearnan et al. (1984) conclude that it is uncertain whether agoraphobic families differ in stability from other families.

The fact that no prospective studies have yet been conducted makes all conclusions on the role of childhood separation anxiety preliminary. The strongest association between childhood separation and adult psychiatric problems seems to exist with depression (Tennant et al. 1981, 1982). Thus, the relationship between childhood separation anxiety and adult panic attacks is tenuous at this point.

3. Psychophysiological Models of Panic Attacks

3.1 Principles of Psychophysiological Models

Psychophysiological models of panic attacks and panic disorder do not assume that panic is qualitatively distinct from other forms of anxiety. Researchers favoring this approach question that panic attacks are spontaneous. At present, these models are less developed and comprehensive than Klein's model.

Psychophysiological models analyze physiological and psychological components of panic and their interaction. Panic attacks are explained by a positive feedback loop (Lader 1975; Mathews et al. 1981; Goldstein and Chambless 1978; Griez and van den Hout 1984; Beck and Emery 1985; Clark et al. 1985) between bodily symptoms of anxiety and the person's reaction to these symptoms (cf. Breggin 1964). Note that internal cues are considered possible triggers for panic attacks. Cognitive processes such as the appraisal of bodily changes or environmental cues as dangerous or as indicating loss of control are considered to be involved in the exacerbation of anxiety.

Some models make specific statements about the physiological components involved in panic. Most frequently mentioned are hyperventilation and minor cardiovascular or vestibular dysfunctions. A typical example for such an approach is given by Clark et al. (1985). This group focusses on panic attacks that are related to hyperventilation. They suggest that patients prone to these attacks increase their respiratory volume when under stress. A vicious circle of hyperventilation, unpleasant body sensations elicited by changes in the blood chemistry, apprehension in response to these sensations, and further hyperventilation culminates in a panic attack.

Whether these processes lead to panic is probably influenced by a number of mediating variables such as current anxiety level, environmental cues, available explanations for body sensations, uncertainty, perceived control, and available coping strategies. Whether the specific bodily sensations and environmental cues have been associated with anxiety states earlier in the individual's learning history is also important (cf. Breggin 1964; Margraf et al. 1986).

Based on the psychophysiological model of panic, effective psychological treatments for panic attacks have been devised (Goldstein 1982; Bonn et al. 1984; Clark et al. 1985; Sartory 1985; Griez and van den Hout 1984; Chambless et al., in press; Salkovskis et al., in press). Treatment components include respiratory training, exposure to panic symptoms, cognitive therapy, paradoxical intention, relaxation, and strategies to increase vagal tone. In addition, some of the more standard exposure treatment packages for agoraphobia have also focussed directly on panic attacks for a number of years (e.g., Hand et al. 1974; Thorpe et al. 1984). Furthermore, long-term efficacy of exposure treatments for agoraphobics, the majority of whom suffer from panic attacks, has repeatedly been demonstrated for periods up to 9 years (Emmelkamp and Kuipers 1979; Munby and Johnston 1980; McPherson et al. 1980; Burns et al. 1983). However, in these earlier studies panic attacks were not considered a phenomenon separate from phobic anxiety and avoidance, and therefore were not assessed separately.

3.2 Empirical Evidence

3.2.1. Positive Feedback Loops in Panic

The positive feedback loop model assumes that certain unpleasant body sensations are an integral part of panic experiences. There is some evidence that such sensations are usually present before the patient experiences panic. In a recent interview study, Hibbert (1984) found that the most frequently reported sequence of events in panic attacks was the perception of an unpleasant bodily sensation (e.g. sweaty palms, dyspnea, or palpitations), followed by anxious catastrophizing cognitions and the full-blown picture of a panic attack. Similarly, Ley (1985) found that somatic symptoms preceded fear in the majority of patients interviewed. Other evidence shows that panic patients specifically are more aware of anxiety-related somatic events in that they report such events more often than patients with generalized anxiety of the same intensity (Hoehn-Saric 1981, 1982; Anderson et al. 1984; cf. Tyrer 1973, 1976). For reviews quoting studies that show hypochondriacal attitudes in agoraphobic patients with panic attacks see Chambless (1982) and Foa et al. (1984).

A direct test of the positive feedback model is currently underway in our laboratory. Since reactions to body sensations are a central part of the model, we manipulate our subjects' perception of bodily changes experimentally using false heart rate feedback. The heart rate feedback paradigm consists of true binary auditory feedback followed by false feedback of an abrupt heart rate increase (equal to a heart rate increase of 50 bpm over 30 sec). As a control for possible differences in cardiac awareness, we asked subjects to match the rate of a train of tone pigs to their heart rates. Reactions of patients meeting DSM-III criteria for panic disorder or agoraphobia with panic attacks and age and sex-matched normal controls are compared. We assessed self-reported anxiety, heart rate, skin conductance level, systolic and diastolic blood pressure.

Our preliminary findings on 15 patients and 21 controls support the positive feedback model (Ehlers et al. 1985). The great majority of subjects did not recognize the false heart rate feedback as false. In both the patient and control groups, only subjects who believed that the false feedback was accurate responded with significant increases in self-reported anxiety (see Fig. 1). Patients, but not controls, also showed significant increases in physiological arousal in response to false but not to accurate feedback. Repeated measures analyses of variance showed significant Group X Time interactions for all physiological variables. Since patients and controls did not differ on the cardiac awareness task, these results point to a role of cognitive-physiological interactions in panic attacks. They support the view that perceived cardiovascular arousal may act as an internal cue that, together with other factors, triggers or exacerbates panic attacks. Only panic patients showed the pattern necessary for positive

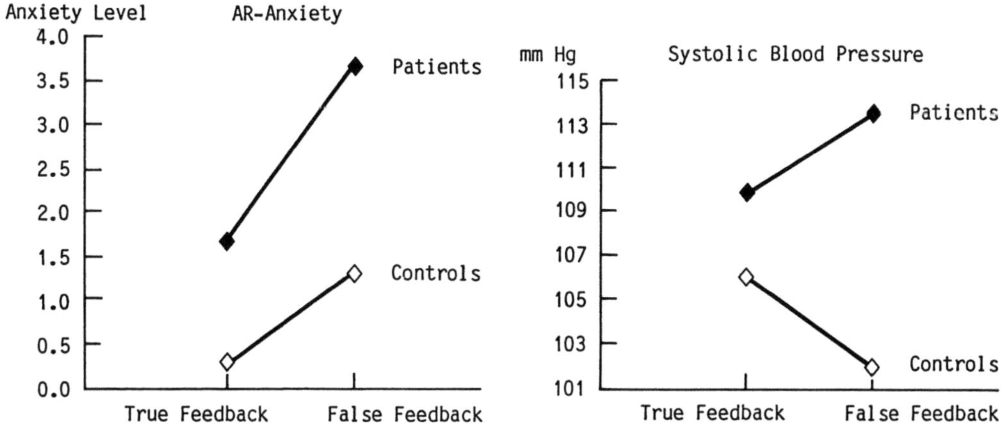

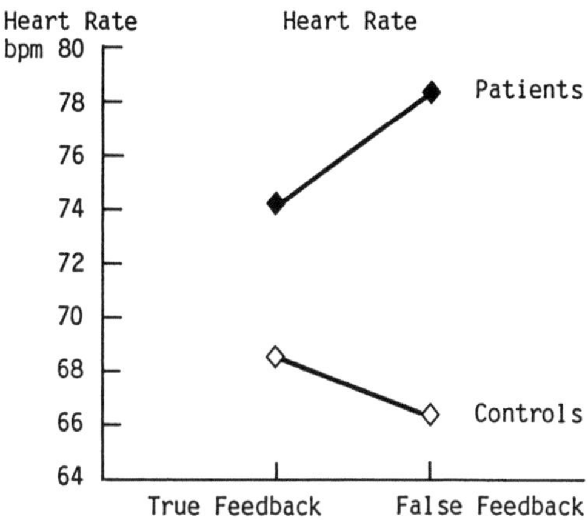

Fig. 1. Responses of panic patients and normal controls to false feedback of a heart rate increase (Ehlers et al. 1985). Results for self-reported anxiety, heart rate, and systolic blood pressure are presented for subjects who did not recognize the false feedback as false. Assessments at the end of a period of true heart rate feedback are compared with those after false feedback. Subjective anxiety was assessed with an Anxiety Rating Scale (AR) ranging from 0 (labelled "none") to 10 (labelled "extreme"). While both patients and controls showed increases in self-reported anxiety, only patients showed increased physiological arousal in response to the false feedback. The same result was found for diastolic blood pressure and skin conductance level

feedback in that they responded to perceived physiological arousal with further increases in arousal.

3.2.2. Role of Cognitions

The role of appraisal processes is supported by evidence that cognitions related to danger are involved in panic attacks. Beck et al.'s (1974) original finding of specific cognitions preceding or accompanying panic attacks or anxiety episodes in all investigated patients was recently replicated by Hibbert (1984). The cognitions reported by panic patients were more centered on death, illness, and loss of control, and were more dramatic, clear, and intrusive than those of patients without panic attacks. This is consistent with the results of Finlay-Jones and Brown (1981) on the specific relevance of "danger" for anxious as opposed to depressed patients.

Furthermore, it has recently been demonstrated that external and internal cues are more likely to be perceived and appraised as threatening by anxious patients. In a series of studies using self-reports and objective measures such as reaction time, Mathews and coworkers showed selective information processing of threat cues in these patients (Butler and Mathews 1983; Mathews and MacLeod 1985, submitted).

3.2.3. Role of Hyperventilation

A number of researchers emphasize the role of hyperventilation in panic attacks and agoraphobia (Lum 1981; Garssen et al. 1983; Bonn et al. 1984; Clark et al. 1985; Ley 1985). Standardized hyperventilation procedures seem to produce symptoms similar or identical to panic attacks in the majority of panic patients (Bonn et al. 1984; Clark et al. 1985). Similar but less intense symptoms were observed in normal controls and other patient groups (Lum 1981; Clark and Hemsley 1982; Thyer et al. 1984). In the study by Bonn et al. (1984) 20 of 21 patients rated the effects of a hyperventilation test as similar to naturally occurring panic attacks, although less intense. However, Gorman et al. (1984) did not find hyperventilation to induce panic. This group used a respiration rate of 30 cycles per minute compared to 60 cycles per minute used by Bonn et al. In addition, there was a sequence confound since voluntary hyperventilation was always preceded by a carbon dioxide inhalation of 20 minutes.

A high resting respiration rate (28 cycles/min) in panic patients was found by Bonn et al. (1984). However, the authors did not report values for the control group. Consistent with the hyperventilation hypothesis, Salkovskis et al. (in press) found significantly lower pCO_2 values at rest in panic patients who rated their attacks as similar to the effects of hyperventilation than in matched normal controls. There were significant correlations between pCO_2 values and the perceived similarity of panic and hyperventilation.

Treatment studies based on this approach in general involved rather small samples but up to two years of follow-up assessments. Both panic frequency and agoraphobic behavior could be controlled or eliminated by a combination of respiration training, cognitive restructuring, and, in some cases, exposure to feared situations (Bonn et al. 1984; Clark et al. 1985; Salkovskis et al., in press). At follow-up, the combination of respiration training and exposure was significantly better than exposure alone (further improvement vs. mild worsening, Bonn et al. 1984). The pCO_2 values were increasingly normalized with successful treatment (Salkovskis et al., in press).

Overall, these results argue strongly in favor of a role for hyperventilation in at least a subgroup of panic attacks. However, it is unclear in what percentage of panic patients hyperventilation may be involved and there are no data regarding hyperventilation in naturally occurring panic attacks.

3.2.4. Role of Cardiovascular Events

Cardiovascular symptoms are reported by nearly all panic patients and number among their most distressing and frequent symptoms. The evidence for measurable cardiovascular dysfunction in panic patients, however, is contradictory. An elevated cardiovascular mortality for male panic patients was found by Coryell et al. (1982). Another recent study did not replicate this finding (Martin et al. 1985; cf. Black et al. 1985). A higher incidence of mitral valve prolapse has been reported in several studies (see Klein and Gorman 1984, for a discussion), but not in others (Hartman et al. 1982; Shear et al. 1984).

The cardiovascular concomitants of panic attacks have recently been studied using ambulatory monitoring. Taylor et al. (1983, in press) and Freedman et al. (1985) found that the majority of panic attacks reported by the patient in diaries were accompanied by clear-cut increases in heart rate. The studies by Taylor et al. demonstrated that these heart rate increases were disproportionate to concurrent activity levels. Panic attacks that were more intense by self-report were more readily identified by heart rate/activity patterns (Taylor et al., in press). EKG monitoring identified the heart rate increases during panic attacks as sinus tachycardias. Taylor et al. also found periods of activity-independent heart rate increases in panic patients that were not associated with panic attacks. These events were less frequent in controls suggesting that patients may be cardiovascularly unstable in some way.

Sartory (1985) has recently developed a therapeutic technique that aims to control sinus tachycardias during panic attacks. In a pilot study, she tought her patients to increase their vagal tone in order to decrease heart rate temporarily. Patient were instructed to use this strategy during panic attacks. Positive therapeutic effects on panic frequency and other anxiety measures were observed.

3.2.5. *Role of Vestibular Dysfunction*

Another possible physiological antecedent for panic attacks are vestibular dysfunctions. These could be important in those panic patients who mainly complain about dizziness and feelings of unsteadiness, two common panic attack symptoms. A pilot study of such patients found a high incidence of abnormal vestibular or auditory function (Jacob et al. 1985). Although no specific neurological disorders were present, 67% of the patients showed positional or spontaneous nystagmus, and pure tone audiograms and acoustic reflexes were abnormal in 26% and 44% of the patients, respectively. Furthermore, 56% had abnormal responses to caloric stimulation, 35% to rotational tests, and 32% to posturography. In another group of patients referred with vestibular disorders and an abnormal response to caloric stimulation, Hood (1975) found a high prevalence of anxiety neurosis (41%). Unfortunately, neither study had a matched control group.

4. Discussion and Conclusions

The 'rediscovery' of panic attacks has had major consequences for the theory and therapy of anxiety disorders. New biologically oriented models (Klein 1981; Sheehan 1982) have drawn needed attention to the special features of panic attacks and the patients suffering from them. However, our review showed that models focussing entirely on the effects of biological and psychological states are not compatible with the majority of the data and with the complexity of the phenomena studied.

The empirical evidence for the biological models' central postulates (Klein 1981; Sheehan 1982) is surprisingly poor. The specificity of drug treatments for panic vs. other types of anxiety has not been supported. Results from so-called panic induction studies do not provide a sufficient empirical basis for Klein's or Sheehan's models. Furthermore, genetic transmission of proneness to panic independent of generalized anxiety has yet to be demonstrated.

The interactive view of psychophysiological models (Lader 1975; Mathews et al. 1981; Beck and Emery 1985; Clark et al. 1985; Margraf et al. 1986) that include the role of cognition and learning seems more able to integrate the data. It is, however, unlikely that any one of the models currently discussed under the header 'psychophysiological' can completely explain the complexities of panic attacks. There are no estimates of the percentage of panic patients whose attacks might be due to any one of the syndromes or mechanisms mentioned above. At this point, the multiplicity of possible mechanisms reduces the explanatory power of any single one. Other mechanisms associated with special disease states would have to be included in any complete theory (MacKenzie and Popkin 1983, McCue and McCue 1984). In any case, the common final pathway by which the different physiological mechanisms lead to panic probably lies in the perception of unpleasant body sensations and their appraisal as dangerous or as indicating loss of control. A first empirical test relevant to the hypothesis of a positive feedback circle between body sensations and response to their perception has been reported here. Panic patients' exaggerated physiological responses to perceived cardiovascular arousal are consistent with the predictions of the psychophysiological model (Ehlers et al. 1985).

The results presented in this chapter have implications for the classification of anxiety disorders. Data supporting psychophysiological models of panic attacks show that it still remains to be determined whether panic attacks are a critical feature in the differential diagnosis of anxiety disorders as DSM-III assumes. The attractiveness of the DSM-III classification depends in part on whether the hypothesis that there are two qualitatively different types of anxiety is confirmed by further evidence. In addition, the clinical application of DSM-III and probably DSM-III-R (Spitzer and Williams 1984; Spitzer 1985) can be problematic since they make distinctions that are not reasonable for every patient and every clinical course (cf. Hallam 1978; Marks 1983; Sheehan and Sheehan 1983; Foa et al. 1984).

The new models of panic attacks have made an important contribution in emphasizing that the attacks themselves should be a focus of treatment. Until recently, most treatment approaches tended to neglect panic attacks even though they are an important source of suffering in anxious patients. Moreover, their alleviation may be crucial for permanent recovery. The efficacy of different therapeutic methods, however, must be determined independently of any inferred etiology of panic attacks. Freedman (1982) has warned that many authors seem to think that a biological (or psychological) cause necessitates a biological (or psychological) therapy. Similarly it is not possible to infer necessary causes from successful treatments. Our review of the literature showed that both drug and psychologically-based treatments seem to be successful in treating panic attacks. More studies are needed that investigate the long-term efficacy of these treatments. Furthermore, information on the characteristics of patients that respond to one or the other form of treatment or their combination is lacking.

5. References

American Psychiatric Assocation (ed) (1980) Diagnostic and statistical manual of mental disorders, 3rd edn. American Psychiatric Press, Washington, D.C.

Anderson DJ, Noyes R, Crowe RR (1984) A comparison of panic disorder and generalized anxiety disorder. Am J Psychiatry 141:572–575

Barlow DH, Cohen AS, Waddell MT, Vermilyea BB, Klosko JS, Blanchard EB, di Nardo PA (1984) Panic and generalized anxiety disorders: Nature and treatment. Beh Ther 15: 431–449

Beck AT, Laude R, Bohnert M (1974) Ideational components of anxiety neurosis. Arch Gen Psychiatry 31:319–325

Beck AT, Emery GD (1985) Anxiety disorders and phobias. A cognitive perspective. Basic Books, New York

Berg I (1976) School phobia in the children of agoraphobic women. Br J Psychiatry 128:86–89

Berg I, Butler A, Pritchard J (1974) Psychiatric illnesses in the mothers of school-phobic adolescents. Br J Psychiatry 125:466–467

Berney T, Kolvin I, Bhate S, Garside R, Jeans J, Kay B, Scarth L (1981) School phobia: A therapeutic trial with clomipramine and short-term outcome. Br J Psychiatry 138:110–118

Black DW, Warrack G, Winokur G (1985) The Iowa Record-Linkage Study. Part III. Excess mortality among patients with 'functional' disorders. Arch Gen Psychiatry 42:82–88

Bonn JA, Readhead CPA, Timmons BA (1984) Enhanced adaptive behavioral response in agoraphobic patients pretreated with breathing retraining. Lancet 1984:665–669

Bowlby J (1969) Attachment and loss. Vol I: Attachment. Basic Books, New York

Bowlby J (1973) Attachment and loss. Vol II: Separation anxiety and anger. Basic Books, New York

Breggin PR (1964) The psychophysiology of anxiety. J Nerv Ment Dis 139:558–568

Brehony KA, Geller ES (1981) Agoraphobia: Appraisal of research and a proposal for an integrative model. In: Hersen M, Eisler R, Miller P (eds) Progress in behavior modification, vol 12. Academic Press, New York

Brown FW (1942) Heredity in the psychoneuroses. Proc R Soc Med 35:785–790

Buglass D, Clarkem J, Henderson AS, Kreitman N, Presley AS (1977) A study of agoraphobic housewives. Psychol Med. 7:73–86

Burns LE, Thorpe GL (1977) Fears and clinical phobias: Epidemiological aspects and the National Survey of Agoraphobics. J Intern Med Res 5 (Supplement 1): 132–139

Burns LE, Thorpe GL, Cavallero A, Gosling J (1983) Agoraphobia eight years after behavioral treatment: A follow-up study with interview, questionnaire and behavioral data. Paper presented at the 17th Annual AABT Convention/World Congress on Behavior Therapy, Washington, D.C.

Butler G, Mathews AM (1983) Cognitive processes in anxiety. Adv Beh Res Ther 5:51–62

Carey G, Gottesman II (1981) Twin and family studies of anxiety, phobic, and obsessive disorders. In: Klein DF, Rabkin J (eds) Anxiety: New research and changing concepts. Raven Press, New York

Carr DB, Sheehan DV (1984) Evidence that panic disorder has a metabolic cause. In: Bal-

lenger JC (ed) Biology of agoraphobia. American Psychiatric Press, Washington, D.C.
Chambless DL (1982) Characteristics of agoraphobics. In: Chambless DL, Goldstein AJ (eds) Agoraphobia: Multiple perspectives on theory and treatment. Wiley, New York
Chambless, DL, Goldstein AJ, Gallagher R, Bright P (in press) Integrating behavior therapy and psychotherapy in the treatment of agoraphobia. Psychotherapy
Chouinard G, Annable L, Fontaine R, Solyom L (1982) Alprazolam in the treatment of generalized anxiety and panic disorders: A double-blind placebo-controlled study. Psychopharmacology 77:229–233
Clark DM, Hemsley DR (1982) The effects of hyperventilation; individual variability and its relation to personality. J Beh Ther Exp Psychiatry 13:41–47
Clark DM, Salkovskis PM, Chalkley AJ (1985) Respiratory control as a treatment for panic attacks. J Beh Ther Exp Psychiatry 16:23–30
Cloninger CB, Martin RL, Clayton P, Guze SB (1981) A blind follow-up and family study of anxiety neurosis: Preliminary analysis of the St. Louis 500. In: Klein DF, Rabkin J (eds) Anxiety: New research and changing concepts. Raven Press, New York
Cohen ME, Badal DW, Kilpatrick A, Reed EW, Whote PD (1951) The high familial prevalence of neurocirculatory asthenia (anxiety neurosis, effort syndrome). Am J Human Gen 3:126–158
Coryell W, Noyes R, Clancy J (1982) Excess mortality in panic disorder. Arch Gen Psychiatry 39:701–703
Crowe RR, Noyes R, Pauls DL, Slymen D (1983) A family study of panic disorder. Arch Gen Psychiatry 40:1065–1069
Ehlers A, Margraf J, Roth WT, Birbaumer N (1985) Received heart rate changes and hyperventilation as anxiety triggers in panic patients. Paper presented at the 15th Annual Meeting of the European Association for Behaviour Therapy, Munich
Emmelkamp PMG, Kuipers A (1979) Agoraphobia: A follow-up study for four years after treatment. Br J Psychiatry 134:352–355
Finlay-Jones R, Brown GW (1981) Types of stressful life event and the onset of anxiety and depressive disorders. Psychol Med 11:801–815
Foa EB, Steketee G, Young MC (1984) Agoraphobia: Phenomenological aspects, associated characteristics, and theoretical considerations. Clin Psychol Review 4:431–457
Freedman DX (1982) Science in the service of the ill. Am J Psychiatry 139:1087–1095
Freedman RB, Ianni P, Ettedgui E, Puthezhath N (1985) Ambulatory monitoring of panic disorder. Arch Gen Psychiatry 42:244–248
Freud S (1895 a) Über die Berechtigung von der Neurasthenie einen bestimmten Symptomenkomplex als 'Angstneurose' abzutrennen. Neurologisches Zentralblatt 2. Also in: Freud S (1952) Gesammelte Werke. Band I. Imago, London, pp 315–342
Freud S (1985 b) Obsessions et phobies. Revenue Neurologique 3. Also in: Freud S (1952) Gesammelte Werke. Band I. Imago, London, pp 345–355
Garssen B, van Veenendaal W, Bloemink R (1983) Agoraphobia and the hyperventilation syndrome. Beh Res Ther 21:643–649
Gittelman-Klein R (1975) Psychiatric characteristics of the relatives of school phobic children. In: Sankar A (ed) Mental health in children, vol I. PDJ Publications, Westbury
Gittelman-Klein R, Klein DF (1973) School phobia: Diagnostic considerations in the light of imipramine effects. J Nerv Ment Dis 156:199–215
Gittelman-Klein R, Klein DF (1980) Separation anxiety in school refusal and its treatment with drugs. In: Hersov A, Berg I (eds) Out of school. Wiley, London
Gittelman-Klein R, Klein DF (1984) Relationship between separation anxiety and panic and agoraphobic disorders. Psychopathology 17 (Supplement):56–65
Goldstein AJ (1982) Agoraphobia: Treatment successes, treatment failures, and theoretical implications. In: Chambless DL, Goldstein AJ (eds) Agoraphobia: Multiple perspectives on theory and treatment. Wiley, New York
Goldstein AJ, Chambless DL (1978) A reanalysis of agoraphobia. Beh Ther 9:47–59
Gorman JM, Askanazi J, Liebowitz MR, Fyer AJ, Stein J, Kinney JM, Klein DF (1984) Response to hyperventilation in a group of patients with panic disorder. Am J Psychiatry 141:857–861
Griez E, van den Hout MA (1984) Carbondioxide and anxiety. Thesis, Rijksuniversiteit, Maastricht
Grunhaus L, Gloger S, Weissturb E (1981) Panic attacks. A review of treatments and pathogenesis. J Nerv Ment Dis 169:608–613
Hallam RS (1978) Agoraphobia: A critical review of the concept. Br J Psychiatry 133:314–319
Hand I, Lamontagne Y, Marks IM (1974) Group exposure (flooding) in vivo for agoraphobics. Br J Psychiatry 124:588–602
Harris EL, Noyes R, Crowe RR, Chaundhry DR (1983) Family study of agoraphobia. Report of a pilot study. Arch Gen Psychiatry, 40:1061–1064
Hartman N, Kramer R, Brown T, Deveraux RB (1982) Panic disorder in patients with mitral valve prolapse. Am J Psychiatry 139:669–670

Hibbert GA (1984) Ideational components of anxiety. Br J Psychiatry 144:618–624

Hoehn-Saric R (1981) Characteristics of chronic anxiety patients. In: Klein DF, Rabkin J (eds) Anxiety: New research and changing concepts. Raven Press, New York

Hoehn-Saric R (1982) Comparison of generalized anxiety disorder with panic disorder patients. Psychopharmacol Bull 18:104–108

Hood DJ (1975) The definition of vestibular habituation. In: Nauton RF (ed) The vestibular system. Academic Press, New York

Jacob R, Moller MB, Turner SM, Wall C (1985) Otoneurological examination of panic disorder and agoraphobia with panic attacks: A pilot study. Am J Psychiatry 142:715–720

Keefe P, Agras WS (1983) Letter to the editor. N Engl J Med 308:341

Klein DF (1964) Delineation of two drug-responsive anxiety syndromes. Psychopharmacologia 5:397–408

Klein DF (1981) Anxiety reconceptualized. In Klein DF, Rabkin J (eds) Anxiety: New research and changing concepts. Raven Press, New York

Klein DF (1984) Psychopharmacological treatment of panic disorder. Psychosomatics 25 (Supplement):32–36

Klein DF, Fink M (1962) Psychiatric reaction patterns to imipramine. Am J Psychiatry 119:432–438

Klein DF, Gorman JM (1984) Panic disorder and mitral valve prolapse. J Clin Psychiatry Monograph 2:14–17

Lader M (1975) The psychophysiology of mental illness. Routledge and Kegan Paul, London

Leckman JF, Weissman MM, Merinkangas KR, Pauls DL, Prusoff BA (1983) Panic disorder and major depression. Arch Gen Psychiatry 40:1055–1060

Ley R (1985) Agoraphobia, the panic attack and the hyperventilation syndrome. Beh Res Ther 23:79–81

Lum LC (1981) Hyperventilation and anxiety state. J Royal Soc Med 74:1–4

MacKenzie TB, Popkin MK (1983) Organic anxiety syndrome. Am J Psychiatry 140:342–344

Margraf J, Ehlers A, Roth WT (1986) Sodium lactate infusions and panic attacks: A review and critique. Psychosomatic Medicine, 48:23–51

Marks I (1983) Are there anticompulsive or antiphobic drugs? Review of evidence. Br J Psychiatry 143:338–347

Martin RL, Cloninger R, Guze SB, Clayton PJ (1985) Mortality in a follow-up of 500 psychiatric outpatients. Arch Gen Psychiatry 42:47–66

Mathews AM, Gelder MG, Johnston DW (1981) Agoraphobia: Nature and treatment. Guilford Press, New York

Mathews AM, MacLeod C (1985) Selective processing of threat cues in anxiety states. Beh Res Ther 23:563–569

Mathews AM, MacLeod C (submitted) Discrimination of threat cues without awareness in anxiety states

Matuzas W, Glass RM (1983) Treatment of agoraphobia and panic attacks. Arch Gen Psychiatry 40:220–222

McCue EC, McCue PA (1984) Organic and hyperventilatory causes of anxiety-type symptoms. Behavioural Psychotherapy 12:308–317

McInnes RG (1937) Observations on heredity in neurosis. Proc Royal Soc Med 30:895–904

McPherson FM, Brougham I, McLaren S (1980) Maintenance of improvement for agoraphobic patients treated by behavioral methods – four year follow-up. Beh Res Ther 18:150–152

Mendel JGC, Klein DF (1969) Anxiety attacks with subsequent agoraphobia. Compr Psychiatry 10:190–195

Moran C, Andrews G (1985) The familial occurrence of agoraphobia. Br J Psychiatry 146:262–267

Munby M, Johnston DW (1980) Agoraphobia: The long-term follow-up of behavioural treatment. Br J Psychiatry 137:418–427

Noyes R, Clancy J, Crowe R, Hoenk PR, Slymen DJ (1978) The familial prevalence of anxiety neurosis. Arch Gen Psychiatry 35:1057–1059

Noyes R, Anderson D, Clancy J, Crowe R, Slymen D, Ghoneim M, Hinrichs J (1984) Diazepam and propanolol in panic disorder and agoraphobia. Arch Gen Psychiatry 41:287–292

Pohl RP, Berchou R, Rainey JM (1982) Tricyclic antidepressants and monoamine oxidase inhibitors in the treatment of agoraphobia. J Clin Psychopharmacol 2:399–407

Raskin M, Peeke HVS, Dickman W, Pinsker H (1982) Panic and generalized anxiety disorders. Arch Gen Psychiatry 39:687–689

Roth M (1984) Agoraphobia, panic disorder and generalized anxiety disorder: Some implications of recent advances. Psychiatric Developments 2:31–52

Salkovskis PM, Jones DRO, Clark DM (in press) Respiratory control in the treatment of panic attacks: Replication and extension with concurrent measurement of behaviour and pCO_2. Brit J Psych

Sartory G (1985) Vagal innervation techniques in the treatment of panic attacks. Paper presented at the 15th Annual Meeting of the European Association of Behaviour Therapy, Munich

Scott JP, Stewart JM, DeGhett VJ (1973) Separation in infant dogs. Emotional response and motivational consequences. In: Scott JP, Senay EC (eds) Separation and depression:

Clinical and research aspects. American Association for the Advancement of Science, Washington, D.C.

Shader R, Goodman M, Gever J (1982) Panic disorders: Current perspectives. J Clin Psychopharmacol 2 (Supplement): 2–10

Shear MK, Devereux RB, Kramer-Foz R, Mann JJ, Frances A (1984) Low prevalence of mitral valve prolapse in patients with panic disorder. Am J Psychiatry 141: 302–303

Sheehan DV (1982) Panic attacks and phobias. N Engl J Med 307: 156–158

Sheehan DV, Sheehan KH (1983) The classification of phobic disorders. Int J Psychiat Med 12: 243–266

Slater E, Shields J (1969) Genetical aspects of anxiety. Br J Psychiatry, Special Publication 3: 62–71

Solyom L, Beck P, Solyom C, Hugel R (1974) Some etiological factors in phobic neurosis. Can Psychiatric Ass J 19: 69–78

Spitzer RL, Williams JB (1984) Diagnostic dilemmas. Psychosomatics 25 (Supplement): 16–20

Spitzer RL (1985) DSM-III-R, draft of October 5, 1985

Suomi SJ, Seaman SF, Lewis JK, Delizio RD, McKinney WT (1978) Effects of imipramine treatment of separation-induced social disorders in rhesus monkeys. Arch Gen Psychiatry 35: 321–325

Taylor CB, Telch MJ, Havvik D (1983) Ambulatory heart rate changes during panic attacks. J Psychiatr Res 17: 261–266

Taylor CB, Sheikh J, Agras WS, Roth WT, Margraf J, Ehlers A, Maddock RJ, Gossard D (in press) Self-report of panic attacks: Agreement with heart rate changes. Am J Psychiatry

Tearnan BH, Telch MJ, Keefe P (1984) Etiology and onset of agoraphobia: A critical review. Compr Psychiatry 25: 51–62

Telch MJ, Tearnan BH, Taylor CB (1983) Antidepressant medication in the treatment of agoraphobia: A critical review. Beh Res Ther 21: 505–517

Telch MJ, Agras WS, Taylor CB, Roth WT, Gallen CC (1985) Combined pharmacological and behavioral treatment for agoraphobia. Beh Res Ther 21: 505–517

Tennant C, Hurry J, Bebbington P (1982) The relation of childhood separation experiences to adult depressive and anxiety states. Br J Psychiatry 141: 475–482

Tennant C, Smith A, Bebbington P, Hurry J (1981) Parental loss in childhood. Relationship to adult psychiatric impairment and contact with psychiatric services. Arch Gen Psychiatry 38: 309–314

Thorpe GL, Burns LE, Smith PJ, Blier MJ (1984) Agoraphobia: Research developments and clinical implications. In Franks CM (ed) New developments in behavior therapy: From research to clinical application. Haworth Press, New York

Thyer BA, Papsdorf JD, Wright P (1984) Physiological and psychological effects of acute intentional hyperventilation. Beh Res Ther 22: 587–590

Torgersen S (1983) Genetic factors in anxiety disorders. Arch Gen Psychiatry 40: 1085–1089

Tyrer PJ (1973) Relevance of bodily feelings in emotion. Lancet 1973: 915–916

Tyrer PJ (1976) The role of bodily feelings in anxiety. Oxford University Press, London

Uhde TW, Boulenger JP, Roy-Byrne PP, Geraci MF, Vittone BJ, Post RM (1985) Longitudinal course of panic disorder: Clinical and biological considerations. Progr Neuro-Pharmacol Biol Psychiatry 9: 39–51

Wheeler EO, White PD, Reed E, Cohen ME (1948) Familial incidence of neurocirculatory asthenia ("anxiety neurosis", "effort syndrome"). J Clin Invest 27: 562

5. Experimental Panic: Biobehavioral Notes on Empirical Findings

Marcel A. van den Hout and Eric Griez

1. Introduction

In order to better understand complex natural phenomena, it is useful to recreate the phenomenon in question under controlled laboratory conditions. Although laboratory models may never be the real thing, they can provide scientists with new ideas and stimulate new research.

For this reason, several efforts were made to reproduce acute panic attacks. Typically, groups of panic patients were compared to controls with respect to their reactions to various, supposedly anxiogenic, pharmacological interventions. While biologically-oriented scientists focussed their attention on non-situational panic, laboratory models of phobic anxiety were also elaborated upon. The latter, however, was generally carried out by stimulus-response psychologists and their models of phobia did not result from pharmacological interventions but rather from manipulating stimulus contingencies.

Although this chapter is devoted to panic, we will first briefly discuss models of phobias. This is not only to demonstrate, in a general sense, the power of experimental psychopathology, but also to show that experimental analysis of phobias may be directly relevant to understanding natural or artificial panic.

In discussing models of phobias and panic, empirical data will be presented that underscores the earlier statement that models are not substitutes for natural phenomena. Although changing some stimulus conditions may produce phobic behavior, it would be wrong to assume that biological factors are of little or no importance. Similarly, it will be argued that, while panic symptoms can be induced by certain pharmacological interventions, it would be wrong to conclude that panic disorder "is" a biological disorder to which behavioral data are of limited or no significance.

This paper touches upon such classical dichotomies as biological vs. psychological and endogenous vs. exogenous. Rather than rephrasing theoretical arguments about the unfruitfulness of such dichotomies, it will be argued that unequivocal data from the very field of experimental psychopathology of anxiety empirically shows that simple "endogenous vs. exogenous" etc. splits should be abandoned when it comes to explaining the complexities of human psychopathology.

2. Phobias

2.1. Some Behavioral Models

For the present purposes, a behavioral model of phobia is defined as any set of manipulations of stimulus contingencies that induce, maintain, and/or reverse phobic behaviour.

From the voluminous work carried out in this area (see, for example, Abramson and Seligman 1977), a suitable example was selected, namely, Baum's experiments on rats (Baum 1970, 1972a–b, 1973, 1976). Cages were constructed that contained a grid floor that could be used to deliver shocks to the rats and a safety ledge to which the animals could jump in order to avoid contact with the conditioned stimulus (CS) (the grid floor) and the unconditioned stimulus (the electrical shock). Delivering shocks a few seconds after the rats were placed on the grid floor quickly produced avoidance behavior, i.e. jumping to the ledge. Reminiscent of the irrationality of phobic fears was the persistence of avoidance behavior even when shocks were no longer given. This would seem to suggest that, in both men and rats, avoidance of an anxiety-provoking situation reduces anxiety and, moreover, that anxiety reduction reinforces avoidance behavior, even in situations where it is no longer even necessary. The resemblance to human phobias becomes even more apparent where treatment is concerned. Removal of the safety ledge prevented any effective conditioned stimulus avoidance and exposed the rats to the "fearful" stimuli. Such exposure *in vivo* resulted primarily in restlessness and in futile efforts to jump to the removed ledge but avoidance efforts extinguish. Strong shocks took approximately 30 minutes to extinguish avoidance; mild shocks, only 3 to 5 minutes. Extinction was facilitated (Baum 1973) by shortening the time interval between CS exposures (cf. massed practice), by having rats observing non-fearing fellows or rats undergoing the same procedure (cf. modelling procedures) and by forcing the animals to explore the grid floor cage (cf. concentrating on the objective environment as a coping skill to handle agoraphobic panic).

Baum's work thus illustrates how changing environmental cues may produce, maintain and/or reverse "phobic" avoidance in rats. The last two points are particularly interesting, as there is such an obvious resemblance to human phobias; indeed it is likely that anxiety-reduction resulting from avoidance is a powerful maintaining factor, both in experimental phobias of rats and in clinical phobias and compulsions (Rachman and Hedgson 1980). As for reversing phobic avoidance, it has been demonstrated time and again that prolongued exposure *in vivo* is an effective treatment approach to situational anxiety (Emmelkamp 1982).

Does this prove that biological determinants play no role in experimental or clinical phobias?

2.2. Biological Aspects of Behavioral Models of Phobias

Rhesus monkeys reared in the laboratory do not appear to get upset when confronted with real or toy snakes; those reared in the wild, however, do. They show clear signs of emotional disturbance and display persistent avoidance behavior (Mineka et al. 1980). Previously non-snake-fearing, laboratory-raised monkeys were made to observe the reaction of their parents, who had been raised in the wild, to simultaneously presented neutral and snake stimuli. One observation of the snake-fearing parental model was all that was needed to induce "fear" and avoidance in the laboratory-raised offspring (Mineka et al. 1983).

One could conclude then that snake phobias in rhesus monkeys are sometimes acquired vicariously; they may also be difficult to extinguish. An attempt was made at reducing avoidance behavior by enabling hungry monkeys to take food only from a box containing a toy snake. "Anxious" behavior, however, persisted across the seven flooding sessions and, at follow-up, 6 months after this exposure therapy, monkeys had relapsed (Mineka and Keir 1983).

It appears that although fear of snakes, within this species, is a learned reaction, it can, to some extent, be unlearned by exposure *in vivo:* it also appears that rhesus monkeys are equipped with some biologically (i.e. genetically) prepared readiness to easily acquire, but not easily lose, snake-fearing reactions. Of course, from an evolutionary perspective, this pattern makes good sense. Might this also be true for human phobias?

In a long series of experiments, Ohman et al. tested the hypotheses (Seligman 1971) that common phobic fears concern dangers that specifically directed our evolution. Subjects who feared/avoided specific natural dangers were supposedly "rewarded" with increased opportunities of survival/reproduction, and, through natural selection, our species is believed to have become equipped with a "preparedness" to easily acquire, but not easily extinguish, fears related to survival.

There is some experimental evidence regarding this "preparedness" that points to human biological equipment as being comparable to that of Mineka's rhesus monkeys. Extinction of electrodermal responses that were classically conditioned by administering a mild electric shock as an unconditioned stimulus was slower when the C.S. was a slide of snakes or spiders than when it was a slide of houses (Ohman et al. 1975). Extinction occurred faster with ontogenetically relevant stimuli (broken electrical chords or equipment) then with phylogenetically relevant slides of spiders or snakes (Hugdahl and Kärker 1981). The effect of observing fearful models on the acquisition of electrodermal fear responses was greater when the C.S. was a slide of an animal such as a spider, snake or rat than when it was of "neutral objects" like flowers, mushrooms, or berries (Hygge and Ohman 1978). Threatening that next slides would be followed by electrical shocks had stronger effects in case of fear relevant pictures (Hugdahl 1978; Kartsonis and Pickersgill 1981). On the other hand, informing previously conditioned subjects that slides would no longer be followed by shocks clearly affected the galvanic skin reaction to neutral slides but electrodermal reactions to fear relevant pictures were not affected. (For an overview, see Hugdahl and Kärker 1981.)

Reviewing some of the work of Baum et al., Mineka et al., and Ohman et al., it appears that by changing environmental cues, phobic reactions can be induced and reduced in rats, monkeys, and men. At the same time, it appears that the biological endowment of the subjects studied is a crucial variable. Phobic responses apparently reflect a closely interwoven complex of interacting causes of both a biological and an environmental nature.

3. Panic

3.1 Biological Models

Beginning in 1919, possible anxiomimetic effects of adrenergics were studied in controls and patients. Yet, interpretation of these older studies has been seriously hampered by the unclear definition of the patient groups. Moreover, the "adrenaline" administered was, in fact, a combination of adrenaline and nor-adrenaline. After a review of the various studies, Guttmacher et al. (1983) tentatively concluded that noradrenaline induce few anxiety symptoms and that adrenaline may be somewhat more effective in inducing anxiety symptoms. Sympaticomimetics do not appear to induce specific psychopathological phenomena and effects on patients and controls appear to be roughly the same. A possible exception is the alpha 2 antagonist yohimbine that in panic patients appeared to have rather specific effects on subjective anxiety and urine MHPG (Charney et al. 1984).

Recently, due to the DSM-III delineation of panic disorder as a separate diagnostic entity, there has been an upsurge of interest in Pitts and McClures (1967) placebo-controlled finding that intravenous infusion of sodium lactate produce more physical anxiety symptoms in panic patients than in normal controls. The study also revealed that panic patients become considerably more distressed by subjective anxiety than do controls.

Lactate infusion seems to be an inspiring biological model of panic. At least 14 replication studies have been published. Three studies lacked a control group (Haslam 1974; Gorman et al. 1983; Gorman et al. 1984a), 8 used normal control subjects (Appleby et al. 1981; Bonn et al. 1971; Fink et al. 1970; Freedman et al. 1984; Kelly et al. 1971; Liebowitz et al. 1984; Rifkin et al. 1981), and 3 used non-panicking neurotics as controls (Gorman et al. 1985; Lapierre et al. 1984; Liebowitz et al. 1985). Panic patients apparently suffer more subjective anxiety during the intervention than do controls. Though it is hazardous to state precisely when anxiety is high enough to warrant the label "panic", it is rather consistently reported that a majority of panic patients and a minority of normal controls experience actual panic. Incidence of lactate induced panic in non-panicking neurotic controls was 2 out of 13 generalized anxiety disorder patients (Lapierre et al. 1984), 1 out of 7 obsessive-compulsives (Gorman et al. 1985), and 1 out of 15 social phobics (Liebowitz et al. 1985).

How does lactate infusion produce its effects? Commenting on Pitts and McClure's work, Grosz and Farmer (1972) explained that sodium lactate is, mole-for-mole, converted into bicarbonate and that lactate infusion thus induces a metabolic alkalosis. The same authors demonstrated that, in controls, the interoceptive changes occurring with lactate and bicarbonate infusion are closely correlated (Grosz and Farmer, 1972). Recently, Liebowitz offered a direct demonstration of the role of sodium lactate in the acid-base balance: pCO_2 decreases while bicarbonate and pH increase (Liebowitz et al. 1985).

Sodium lactate infusion is not the only intervention that reliably and specifically reproduces panic phenomena. The lactate-induced hypocapnia and alkalosis, as well as the accompanying subjective sensations, are reminiscent of the effects of single inhalations of 35% CO_2/65% O_2. One vital capacity inhalation of the mixture results in an alveolar hypercapnia with a violent stimulation of the chemoregulatory system that immediately intensifies ventilation. Alveolar pCO_2 displays a rapid fall and resulting in a hypocapnic undershoot (van den Hout and Griez 1985). The alveolar changes are reflected in comparable phenomena in the arterial plasma: a hypercapnic acidosis is followed by a pCO_2 drop/pH rise, resulting in a hypocapnic alkalosis. During the changes in blood gases, electrolyte changes are apparent: a biphasic change in ionized calcium (an initial rise followed by a beneath base-line drop) and an inverted U pattern of potassium (Griez and van den Hout 1984). Cardiovascular effects are largely sympaticomimetic (Griez and van den Hout 1983a).

These physiological changes are accompanied by distinct somatic sensations, that are highly comparable to those occurring during natural or lactate induced panic. In normal subjects these sensations can be reduced by approximately 20% by premedication with 60 mg of propranolol (van den Hout and Griez 1984).

As for subjective anxiety, normal subjects were hardly affected by CO_2 inhalation (Griez and van den Hout 1982; van den Hout and Griez 1982a). Panic patients, on the other hand, consistently show quite high anxiety during CO_2 challenge (Griez et al. 1985). Though panic patients also show somewhat higher anxiety during placebo (inhalation of air), the different reactions of panic patients and normal controls cannot statistically be accounted for by a difference in general or "background" anxiety levels as reflected by placebo scores (van den Hout et al. 1985).

Results from studies on lactate infusion, bicarbonate infusion, and CO_2 inhalation point to pH changes as a physiological concomitant in the genesis of experimentally induced panic. Further support for acid-base changes underlying these panicomimetics comes from the hyperventilation literature (cf. Garssen et al. 1983; Lum 1981; Clark and Salkovskis 1985).

It has been proposed that panic disorder is a biological disorder (Carr and Sheehan 1984) and, in line with the experimental findings cited above, hypotheses were investigated concerning possible underlying pathophysiological abnormalities in acid-base regulation and chemo-regulatory CO_2

sensitivity in panic patients. The data, however, is inconclusive. Although rest-hypocapnia was observed in some studies (Folgering and Colla 1978), other researchers reported normal pCO_2 levels (Weiman 1968; Hardonk and Beumer 1979), while still others observed incidental hypercapnia in panic patients (Fried et al. 1984; Gorman et al. 1985). Chemoregulatory CO_2 hypersensitivity may not be characteristic of hyperventilation patients; if anything, a hyposensitivity is more likely (Pearson 1985). It has recently been speculated that perhaps the C.N.S. has "suffocation receptors" acting upon the locus coeruleus and maybe panic patients suffer from a hypersensitivity of these suffocation receptors (Gorman et al. 1984b). These speculations are interesting but will be difficult to test.

By way of summary, it appears that, in vulnerable subjects, panic symptoms can be reproduced by lactate infusion or CO_2 inhalation. As far as an *explanation* of this lactate/CO_2 effect is concerned, one may postulate underlying pathophysiological mechanisms. Indeed, identification and clarification of such possible biological abnormalities warrant further study. For the time being, however, there is no a-priori reason whatsoever to assume that in the explanation of lactate/CO_2 effects, pathophysiological accounts should take preference to behavioral or cognitive ones.

3.2. Behavioral Aspects of Pharmacological Panic Models

The most parsimonious behavioral account of recurrent panic attacks may be the following. Innocuous environmental cues may trigger phobic anxiety reactions in some people. Likewise, it can be hypothesized that some people may become frightened by the perception of certain harmless bodily sensations. More specifically, it may be assumed that panic patients constitute the subgroup of interoceptive phobics whose phobic fear is triggered by the perception of those bodily sensations which also happen to be part of the anxiety response. Both clinical impressions and preliminary controlled data from our laboratory suggest that interoceptive fears typically concern the subset of interoceptive sensations that arise when the proper functioning of vital organ systems is at stake. Both palpitations and paresthesias are common in panic patients. The fact that they often express intense anxiety for palpitations but rarely for paresthesias, may indicate that some prepared learning also takes place in the realm of interoceptive stimuli.

As in the case of situational phobias (Marks 1978), a fully clarified pathogenesis may not be needed before one can assume that conditioning processes play a role in the maintenance of panic (Ackerman and Sachar 1974).

The idea that fear of fear underlies panic disorder is far from new (e.g. Evans 1972; Clark and Salkovskis 1984; Griez and van den Hout 1984; Margraf et al., see chapter 4; Eysenck 1968), and the above considerations are merely a shorthand, behavioral reformulation of the age-old belief that people may become fearful of fear itself. From this fear of fear model, some inferences can be drawn that are of interest when it comes to explaining lactate and CO_2 effects. Far from being incompatible with biological approaches, behavioral data may enhance the validity of lactate or CO_2 panic models.

1. A first prediction is that *artificial provocation of bodily anxiety symptoms will result in subjective anxiety in panic patients but not in normal subjects and not in non-panic stricken neurotic controls.* The lactate and CO_2 literature reviewed above strongly supports this inference (Ackerman and Sachar 1974; Griez et al. 1985). Nevertheless, this prediction is somewhat post hoc and appears to be a postdiction. Also, the very same prediction will be made by many who favor a physicodeterministic view of panic.

2. A second inference would be that the *reported affective changes in lactate or CO_2 challenges can to some extend be controlled by environmental or cognitive/instructional variables.*

To our knowledge, no experiment on lactate has been published that addresses this issue. It is noteworthy, however, that, in lactate trials, a large number of panic patients report that the mere presence of the experimenter is reassuring enough to prevent full-blown panic (Bonn et al. 1971; Kelly et al. 1971).

This is in line with our CO_2 inhalation experiences with patients. In normal subjects, it was found that subjective CO_2 effects can be manipulated by only slightly changing the experimental instruction. Those subjects who expected pleasant subjective states reported the same, while those who expected unpleasant experiences reported distress. This instruction-effect was significantly lower when a placebo (air) was administered (van den Hout and Griez 1982b). It appears that in panic patients too, the affective effects of CO_2 can be influenced by changing the instructional set (Rapee 1985).

3. Repeated and prolongued exposure *in vivo* reduces phobic fears. If panic disorder represents an introceptive fear that can be induced by CO_2 or lactate, it should be expected *that repeated and prolongued administrations of lactate or CO_2 to vulnerable individuals produces less anxiety as the number/duration of administrations increases.* Bonn et al. (1975), using lactate infusion induced maximum anxiety in 33 anxiety neurotics during 6 twenty minute sessions, and found that "the phobophobic element which was so frequently elicited from these patients was substantially reduced. In a recent CO_2 study, 13 panic patients and 8 controls received a series of 35% CO_2/65% O_2 inhalations (6 sessions; 10 inhalations per session) as well as air inhalation (3 sessions; 10 inhalations per session). The order was CO_2 (3 sessions), air (3 sessions), CO_2 (3 sessions) or air (3 sessions), CO_2 (3 sessions), CO_2 (3 sessions). There was a clear habituation effect in the patient group. In the CO_2-air-CO_2 condition, mean subjective anxiety scores – expressed on a 100 point rating scale – were: 56/47/43, 8/12/6, 46/41/28. Scores in the air-CO_2-CO_2 condition were: 20/7/8, 62/52/36, 24/19/17. Normals did not report any distress after air and only very little, quickly disappearing anxiety after CO_2 inhalation.

4. Exposure *in vivo* for situational phobias not only reduces fear/avoidance of the situations involved in the treatment program, but also typically causes generalisation.

An intriguing inference from accounting for CO_2/lactate effects in terms of interoceptive phobia is that *repeated/prolongued exposure to CO_2 or lactate improves the clinical condition of the patient.*

As for lactate, Bonn et al.'s (1971) aforementioned 6 sessions of 20-minute intravenous infusions with 33 panic patients resulted in a clinical improvement. Numerous cases were reported allegedly demonstrating the beneficial effects of CO_2 inhalation in the treatment of neurosis (Meduna, 1955). The theoretical rationale of these uncontrolled findings seems somewhat outdated these days. The techniques consisted of a long series of subsequent inhalations, often resulting in coma, while outcome data were uncontrolled and the indication was rather non-specific. The positive effects of this broad spectrum type of CO_2 therapy were not confirmed in later trials (Harris 1954; Hawkins and Tibetts 1956). Very little is known about the effects of a series of single, non coma, CO_2 inhalations in the treatment of panic states, however; two successful cases have been published (Latimer 1977; Griez and van den Hout 1983b). In a crossover design with 14 panic patients, the panic-reducing effects of propranolol (Noyes et al. 1981) were compared with those of 35% CO_2 inhalation. CO_2 produced a significant reduction of fear of autonomic panic sensations, state- and trait anxiety, agoraphobic anxiety and avoidance, and of the frequency of panicking; propranolol resulted in improvements in state- and agoraphobic anxiety. Except for trait anxiety, CO_2 was superior on all measures, most clearly so on fear of autonomic panic sensations. At the 6-month follow-up, 3 patients required further treatment. Except for state anxiety, improvements were, on the average, maintained (Griez and van den Hout 1985).

5. A last inference would be that *successful treatment of panic, be it by pharmacological or psychological means, will reduce the vulnerability to CO_2 or lactate.*

No data is available on changing CO_2 vulnerability through treatment, apart from the studies discussed above (van den Hout et al. 1985; Griez and van den Hout 1985). In the case of lactate, it has been shown that successful treatment with anti-depressants (MAO inhibitors or tricyclics) reduces lactate vulnerability (Kelly et al. 1971; Rifkin et al. 1981; Fyer et al. 1985). Of particular current interest is the recent case history by Guttmacher and Nelles (1984) of a patient who lost her lactate vulnerability after a successful behavioral treatment for her anxiety complaints.

4. Concluding Remarks

It has been argued that the very fact that certain pharmacological agents induce panic in vulnerable individuals indicates that, in some way, panic disorder is ultimately a biological disorder (Carr and Sheehan 1984; Gorman et al. 1985; Sheehan 1982).

This argument is not especially convincing. Just as the psychological nature of simple phobias is not "proved" by the feasability of behavioral lab-models, the lactate or CO_2 effects, in themselves, are not suitable to support any strictly physico-deterministic hypotheses.

A comparable non sequitur would be that the efficiency of biological vs. psychological interventions demonstrates the nature of the pathogenesis. Short- and long-term effectiveness of *in vivo* exposure in agoraphobia (Emmelkamp et al. 1978; Marks 1971; McPharson et al. 1980; Munby and Johnston 1980), does not tell us that agoraphobia "is" a psychological/behavioural disorder. Likewise, the positive effects of tri-cyclics in panic disorder (or benzodiazepines in acute grief) are far from sufficient to demonstrate that panic disorder (or grief) "are" somatic disorders.

Lewis (1971) argued that, on a theoretical level, the old but persistent Möbian dichotomy of "endogenous versus exogenous" runs into serious conceptual problems and is quite useless. Data from the very realm of experimental psychopathology of neurotic anxiety offers empirical support for Lewis' conclusions. Responses of subjects in laboratory experiments on anxiety seem to reflect interactions between psychological/environmental and biological variables. This holds true for both conditioning models of phobias and pharmacologic models of panic. The observed interactions are highly interesting but fairly complex.

As yet, we do not know their exact nature or in what respects laboratory observations do or do not reflect the dynamics of natural anxiety or panic.

Yet, however, complex the questions and answers of experimental psychopathology may be, we do know that, in the final analysis, we are dealing with empirical issues. A suitable approach to further clarification may consist of interdisciplinary attempts to construct, develop, and validate experimental models of neurotic anxiety.

5. References

Abramson LY, Seligman MEP (1977) Modeling Psychopathology in the Laboratory: History and Rationale. In: Maser JD, Seligman MEP (eds) Psychopathology: Experimental Models. Freeman & Co., San Francisco

Ackerman SH, Sachar EJ (1974) The Lactate Theory of Anxiety: A Review and Reevaluation. Psychosom Med 36:69–81

Appleby IL, Klein DF, Sachar EJ, Levitt M (1981) Biochemical Indices of Lactate-Induced Panic: A Preliminary Report. In: Klein DF, Rabkin J (eds) Anxiety: New Research and Changing Concepts. Raven Press, New York

Baum M (1970) Extinction of avoidance-responding through response prevention (flooding). Psychol Bull 74:276–280

Baum M (1972a) Flooding (response prevention) in rats: The effects of immediate vs. delayed flooding and of changed illumination conditions during flooding. Canadian J Psych 26:190–195

Baum M (1972b) Repeated acquisition and extinction of avoidance in rats using flooding (response prevention) learning and motivation. 3:272–278

Baum M (1973) Extinction of avoidance in rats:

the effects of chlorpromazine and methylphenidate administered in conjunction with flooding (response-prevention). Beh Res Ther 11:165–173

Baum M (1976) Instrumental learning. In: Feldmann NP, Broadburst A (eds) Theoretical and experimental basis of behavior therapists. John Wiley, New York

Bonn JA, Harrison J, Rees WL (1971) Lactate induced anxiety: therapeutic applications. Brit J Psychiat 199:468–470

Carr DB, Sheehan DV (1984) Panic Anxiety: A new biological model. J Clin Psychiatry 45:323–330

Charney D, Henninger G, Breier A (1984) Nonadrenergic functioning in panic patients. Arch Gen Psychiatry 41:751–763

Clark DM, Salkovskis PM (1985) Cognitive and physiological processes in panic attacks. Paper presented at the 15th Annual Meeting of the European Association for Behaviour Therapy. München

Clark DM, Salkovskis PM (1984) A model for the development of a panic attack. Unpublished paper

Emmelkamp PMG (1982) Phobic and obsessive compulsive disorders: theory, research and practice. Plenum press, New York

Emmelkamp PMG, Kuipers ACM, Eggeraat JB (1978) Cognitive modification versus prolonged exposure in vivo: A comparison with agoraphobics as subjects. Beh Res Ther 16:33–41

Evans IM (1972) A conditioning model of a common fear pattern: fear of fear. Psychotherapy: theory, research and practice 9:238–241

Eysenck HJ (1968) A theory of the incubation of anxiety/fear responses. Beh Res Ther 6:309–321

Fink M, Taylor MA, Volavka J (1970) anxiety precipitated by lactate. New Engl J Med 281:1429

Folgering H, Colla P (1978) Some anomalies in the control of pCO_2 in patients with hyperventilation syndrome. Bull European de Physiopathologie respiratoire 14:503–512

Freedman RR, Ianni P, Ettedgui E, Pohl R, Rainey JM (1984) Psychophysiological factors in panic disorder. Psychopathology supplement 1, 17:66–73

Fried RMC, Fox MC, Carlton RM, Rubin SR (1984) Methods and protocols for assessing hyperventilation and its treatment. J Drug Ther Res 9:280–288

Fyer AJ, Liebowitz M, Gorman J, Davies S, Klein D (1985) Lactate vulnerability of remitted panic patients. Psychiatry Res 14:143–148

Garsen B, van Veenendaal W, Bloemink R (1983) Agoraphobia and the hyperventilation syndrome. Beh Res Ther 21:643–649

Gorman JM, Levy G, Liebowitz M, McGrath P, Appleby I, Dillon D, Davies S, Klein DF (1983) Effect of acute, beta-adrenergic blockade on lactate induced panic. Arch Gen Psychiatry 40:1079–1082

Gorman JM, Liebowitz MR, Fyer A, Ditton D, Davies S, Stein J, Klein DF (1985) Lactate infusions in obsessive-compulsive neurosis. Amer J Psychiat 142:864–866

Gorman JM, Martinez J, Liebowitz M, Fyer A, Klein DF (1984a) Hypoglycemia and panic attacks. Amer J Psychiat 141:857–861

Gorman JM, Askanazi J, Lebowitz MR, Fyer AJ, Stein J, Kinney JM, Klein DF (1984b) Response to hyperventilation in a group of patients with panic disorder. Amer J Psychiat 141:857–861

Griez E, van den Hout MA (1982) Effects of carbondioxide-oxygen inhalations on subjective anxiety and some neurovegetative parameters. J Beh Ther Exp Psychiatry 13:27–32

Griez E, van den Hout MA (1983a) Carbondioxide and anxiety. Cardiovascular effects of a single inhalation. J Beh Ther Exp Psychiatry 14:297–304

Griez E, van den Hout MA (1983b) Treatment of phobophobia by exposure to CO_2 induced anxiety symptoms. J Nerv Ment Dis 171:506–508

Griez E, van den Hout MA (1984) Carbondioxide and anxiety: An experimental approach to a clinical claim. Dissertation, State University of Limburg, Maastricht

Griez E, van den Hout MA (1985) Fear of panic, CO_2 induced exposure vs. beta blocking aided avoidance. Beh Res Ther. Accepted for publication

Griez E, Lousberg H, van den Hout MA, van der Molen GM (1985) CO_2 vulnerability in Panic Disorder. In Press

Grosz HJ, Farmer BB (1969) Blood Lactate in the development of anxiety symptoms. Arch Gen Psychiatry 21:611–619

Grosz HJ, Farmer BB (1972) Pitt's and McClure's Lactate-Anxiety Study Revisited. Brit J Psychiatry 120:415–418

Guttmacher LB, Murphy DL, Insel TR (1983) Pharmacologic Models of Anxiety. Comprehens Psychiat 24:312–326

Guttmacher LB, Nelles C (1984) In vivo desensitization alternation of lactate induced panic: a case study. Beh Ther 15:369–372

Hardonk HJ, Beumer HM (1979) Hyperventilation syndrome. In: Handbook of Clinical Neurology, vol 38. Neurological manifestation of the systemic diseases, part. Vinken IPJ, Bruyne Y (eds), Amsterdam

Harris A (1954) A comparative study of results in neurotic patients treated by two different methods. J Ment Sci 100:718–721

Haslam MT (1974) The Relationship Between the Effect of Lactate Infusion on Anxiety States, and their Amelioration by Carbon Dioxide Inhalation. Brit J Psychiat 125:88–90

Hawkings JR, Tibbits RW (1956) Carbon dioxide inhalation therapy in neurosis: A controlled clinical trial. J Ment Sci 102:52–59

Hout van den MA, Griez E (1982 a) Cardiovascular and subjective responses to inhalation of carbondioxide. Psychother Psychosom 37: 75–82

Hout van den MA, Griez E (1982 b) Cognitive factors in carbon dioxide therapy. J Psychosom Res 26:209–214

Hout van den MA, Griez E (1984) Panic symptoms after inhalation of carbon dioxide. Brit J Psychiat 144:503–507

Hout van den MA, Griez E (1985) Peripheral panic symptoms occur during changes in alveolar carbon dioxide. Comprehens Psychiat 26:381–387

Hugdahl K (1978) Electrodermal conditioning to potentially phobic stimuli: effects of instructed extinction. Behav Res Ther 16:315–321

Hugdahl K, Kärker A (1981) Biological vs. experimental factors in phobic conditioning. Behav Res Ther 19:109–115

Hygge S, Ohman A (1978) Modelling processes in the evolution of fears: vicarious electrodermal conditioning to fear relevant stimuli. J Personality Soc Psychol 36:271–279

Kartsounis LD, Pickersgill MJ (1981) Orienting to stimuli that others fear. Brit J Clin Psychol 20:261–263

Kelly D, Mitchell-Heggs N, Shermann D (1971) Anxiety and the effects of sodium lactate assessed clinically and physiologically. Brit J Psychiat 119:129–141

Lapierre YD, Knott VJ, Gray R (1984) Psychophysiological correlates of sodium lactate. Psychopharmacol Bull 20:50–57

Latimer P (1977) Carbon dioxide as a reciprocal inhibitor in the treatment of neurosis. J Beh Ther Exp Psychiat 8:83–85

Lewis A (1971) 'Endogenous' and 'exogenous': a useful dichotomy? Psychol Med 1:191–196

Liebowitz MR, Fyer AJ, Gorman JM, Pitton D, Appleby IL, Levy GL, Anderson S, Levitt M, Paly M, Sharon O, Davies RN, Klein DF (1984) Lactate Provocation of Panic Attacks: Clinical and behavioral findings. Arch Gen Psychiatry 41:764–770

Liebowitz MR, Fyer A, Gorman J, Pitton D, Davies S, Stein J, Cohen B, Klein DF (1985) Specificity of lactate infusions in social phobia versus panic disorders. Amer J Psychiat 142: 947–950

Liebowitz M, Gorman J, Fyer M, Miller D, Levy S, Appleby I, Anderson S, Paly M, Davies S, Klein DF (1985) Lactate provocation of panic attacks: Biochemical and physiological findings. Arch Gen Psychiatry 42:709–719

Lum LC (1981) Hyperventilation and anxiety state. J Royal Soc Med 7:1–4

Marks IM (1971) Phobic disorders four years after treatment: a prospective follow-up. Brit J Psychiat 118:683–688

McPherson FM, Brougham L, McLaren S (1980) Maintenance of improvement in agoraphobic patients treated by behavioural methods. A four year follow-up. Beh Res Ther 18:150–152

Meduna LJ (ed) (1955) Carbon dioxide therapy: A neurophysiological treatment of nervous disorders. Charles Thomas, Springfield Illinois

Mineka S, Davidson M, Keir R, Cook M (1983) Observational conditioning of snake fear in rhesus monkeys. J Abnorm Psychol 92

Mineka S, Keir R (1983) The effects of flooding on reducing snake fear in rhesus monkeys: Six months follow up and further flooding. Beh Res Ther 21:527–536

Mineka S, Keir R, Price V (1980) Fear of snakes in wild and laboratory reared rhesus monkeys (Macaca mulatta). Anim Learn Beh 8:653–663

Munby M, Johnston DW (1980) Agoraphobia: the long-terms follow-up of behavioural treatment. Brit J Psychiat 137:418–427

Noyes R, Kathol R, Clancey J, Crowe RR (1981) Anti-anxiety effects of propranolol: a review of clinical studies. In: Klein DF, Rabkin J (eds) Anxiety: New research and changing concepts. Raven Press

Ohman A, Eriksson A, Olofsson C (1975) One trial learning and superior resistance to extinction of autonomic responses conditioned to potentially phobic stimuli. J Com Physiol Psychol 88:619–627

Pearson MG (1985) Abnormalities of respiratory centre function and pottassium homeostatis in the chronic hyperventilation syndrom. Paper presented at the Vth International symposium on respiratory psychophysiology. Nijmegen

Pitts FN, McClure JN (1967) Lactate metabolism in anxiety neurosis. New Engl J Med 277:1329 –1336

Rachman S, Hodgson R (1980) Obsessions and compulsions. Prentice Hall, Inc, Englewood Cliffs, New Yersey

Rapee R (1985) Personal communication. Kensington

Rifkin A, Klein DF, Dillon D (1981) Blockade by imipramine or desipramine of panic induced by sodium lactate. Amer J Psychiat 138:676–677

Seligman MEP (1971) Phobias and preparedness. Beh Ther 2:307–320

Sheehan DV (1982) Panic attacks and phobias. New Engl J Med 307:156–158

Weiman S (1968) Das Hyperventilationssyndrom. Urban und Schwarzenberg, München

6. Experimental Induction of Panic Attacks

Anke Ehlers, Jürgen Margraf, and Walton T. Roth

1. Introduction

In the field of anxiety research much attention has recently been focussed on panic attacks. Freedman and Glass (1984) devoted their recent review of progress in psychiatry in the *Journal of the American Medical Association* almost exclusively to this topic. As we discuss in detail in the chapter by Margraf, Ehlers, and Roth in this book, the major impetus for this development has come from the claim that panic is a biologically unique form of anxiety (Klein 1981; Sheehan 1982). This assumption, however, remains controversial (Marks 1983; Foa et al. 1984; Hand 1984).

Support for a qualitative difference of panic anxiety from other forms of anxiety has been seen in the results of so-called 'panic induction' studies. These studies investigate the effects of challenge tests such as infusion of sodium lactate or inhalation of carbon dioxide (CO_2). Several authors have reported that patients suffering from panic attacks, but not normal controls, panic in response to these challenges (Pitts and McClure 1967; Bonn et al. 1971; Fink et al. 1971; Kelly et al. 1971; Appleby et al. 1981; Rifkin et al. 1981; Liebowitz et al. 1984, 1985; Rainey et al. 1984a, 1984b; Gorman et al. 1984a). This led Freedman and Glass (1984) to conclude "Uniquely for psychiatric disorders, anxiety attacks can be readily and safely elicited by biological challenges – CO_2 inhalation, infusion of lactate . . . The essential elements of clinical attacks are elicited by and large only in patients" (p. 2226).

In the study of panic disorder, panic challenge tests could be useful for different

Preparation of this manuscript was supported in part by the Medical Research Service of the Veterans Administration and the Upjohn Company.

purposes. First, they have been proposed as an experimental model for evoking and studying anxiety episodes similar or even identical to natural panic attacks. Such a model could help to gain insights in the pathophysiology of panic attacks and could be used to investigate the efficacy of treatments. Second, some authors suggest that response to lactate or CO_2 is a possible biological marker for panic attacks. For example, Shader et al. (1982) conclude "Biological evidence of the distinctness of panic disorders from other anxiety disorders comes primarily from lactate challenge tests" (p. 4). And Carr and Sheehan (1984, p. 100) infer from the results of panic induction studies "that panic disorder is a biological disease."

In this chapter, we critically discuss the evidence from panic induction studies using lactate infusion and CO_2 inhalation and present our own data. We examine whether response to lactate or CO_2 is suitable for the purposes mentioned above.

2. Sodium Lactate and Carbon Dioxide as Panic Challenges – Historical Development

2.1 Lactate Infusion and Panic Attacks

The first study on lactate infusion and anxiety was conducted by Pitts and McClure in 1967. Based on reports that patients with anxiety neurosis showed excessive lactate production during standard exercise tasks concomitant with anxiety symptoms, Pitts and McClure developed the idea that the lactate ion itself could produce anxiety attacks in susceptible persons. In a double-blind study, they found sodium lactate to produce anxiety attacks in 13 of 14 anxiety neurotics but only in two of 10 normal controls. Subsequent studies confirmed that lactate infusions precipitate anxiety attacks in many patients prone to them. However, Pitts' and McClure's original explanation for lactate's panic-inducing effects was rejected (Elridge 1968; Henderson 1968; Grosz and Farmer 1969, 1972; Levitt 1972; Grosz 1973; Ackerman and Sachar 1974) and interest in the effects of lactate infusions vanished temporarily. With the new focus on panic attacks in anxiety research, several research centers started new studies on lactate infusions (Appleby et al. 1981; Knott et al. 1981; Freedman et al. 1984; Lapierre et al. 1984; Liebowitz et al. 1984, 1985; Rainey et al. 1984b). Contemporary researchers focus more narrowly on panic disorder instead of considering sodium lactate as the biological substrate of anxiety in general (Pitts 1969).

2.2. Carbon Dioxide Inhalation and Panic Attacks

Interest in carbon dioxide inhalation (CO_2) has come from a completely different direction. Early reports that neurotic patients benefited from inhalation of high concentrations of CO_2 (cf. Meduna 1955; Griez and van den Hout 1984), led Wolpe (1958) to assume that CO_2 inhalation could be used therapeutically to inhibit anxiety. He presented case reports in which repeated single inhalation of CO_2 successfully treated non-situational 'pervasive anxiety'. Subsequent studies reported that Wolpe's method indeed led to anxiety reduction (Slater and Levy 1966; Ley and Walker 1973; Haslam 1974). In their attempts to replicate these findings, however, Griez and van den Hout (1984) found in a series of studies that single inhalation of a 35% CO_2/65% oxygen mixture was not anxiety-reducing, neither in normal subjects nor in anxiety patients (Griez and van den Hout 1982; van den Hout and Griez 1982a, 1982b). Instead, two studies in normal volunteers showed sympathicomimetic and anxiomimetic effects (Griez and van den Hout 1983; van den Hout and Griez 1984). CO_2 inhalation appeared to mimic the symptoms of panic attacks quite accurately. Griez and van den Hout (1984) explain Wolpe's therapeutic successes as the result of exposure to anxiety-inducing interoceptive cues provoked by CO_2 (cf. Latimer 1977).

Recently Gorman et al. (1984a) also reported panic induction by CO_2 inhalation. These authors used prolonged inhalation of smaller concentrations of CO_2 (5% CO_2 in room air for 20 min). Seven of twelve panic patients panicked in response to CO_2, a rate equal to that during lactate infusion (eight attacks). The four control subjects studied did not panic. Gorman et al. relate their results to earlier reports of intolerance of CO_2 in patients with 'neurocirculatory asthenia' and 'irritable heart syndrome'.

3. Results of Panic Induction Studies

3.1. Effects of Lactate and CO_2

A detailed review of the effects of lactate infusion is found in Margraf et al. (1986). In this section, we briefly summarize the results of this review and present the findings from CO_2 inhalation studies.

3.1.1. Self-reported Anxiety and Symptoms

In three studies that used standard measures of *anxiety, lactate infusion* was found to induce moderate levels of anxiety in patients and generally lower levels of anxiety in control subjects (Kelly et al. 1971; Rainey et al. 1984a, 1984b; cf. Freedman et al. 1984; Lapierre et al. 1984). For *inhalation of* high *CO_2* concentrations, inconsistent effects on subjective anxiety were reported ranging from decreases to increases (Slater and Levy 1966; Ley and Walker 1973; Haslam 1974; Griez and van den Hout 1982; van den Hout and Griez 1982a, 1982b). Van den Hout and Griez (1982a) demonstrated in normal subjects that the effects of CO_2 on subjective state depended on the expectations set by the instructions.

In five studies that report *lactate-induced symptoms* in panic or anxiety patients, lactate was found to produce various symptoms related to anxiety and distress (Pitts and McClure 1967; Kelly et al. 1971; Bonn et al. 1971; Rifkin et al. 1981; Liebowitz et al. 1984). In all of these studies, the symptoms were significantly more frequent and intense under lactate than under placebo. Lactate effects were stronger in patients than in normal controls in studies that reported values for both groups (Pitts and McClure 1967; Kelly et al. 1971). Still, controls reported a significant number of symptoms under lactate (Pitts and McClure 1967; Kelly et al. 1971; Grosz and Farmer 1972), which were qualitatively comparable to those reported by the patients.

CO_2-induced symptoms were studied by van den Hout and Griez (1984) in normal volunteers. Single inhalation of a 35% CO_2/65% oxygen mixture produced an average of 7.5 of 12 DSM-III (American Psychiatric Association 1980) panic symptoms. Inhalation of room air produced fewer symptoms (1.25). Gorman et al. (1984a) reported that inhalation of 5% CO_2 for 20 min produced 'the full range of common symptoms of panic attacks' in 7 of 12 patients. Symptoms of other patients and controls were not reported.

3.1.2. Physiological Effects

In studies that assessed the *physiological* effects of *lactate infusion,* increases in heart rate, blood pressure, skin conductance level and forearm blood flow were consistently reported (Kelly et al. 1971; Bonn et al. 1971, 1973; Knott et al. 1981; Gorman et al. 1983; Rainey et al. 1984a, 1984b; Freedman et al. 1984; Lapierre et al. 1984; Liebowitz et al. 1985). Non-autonomic indicators of activation ('arousal') such as electromyogram and respiration rate failed to show consistent changes. CNS changes included increased beta and delta and decreased alpha (Fink et al. 1971; Knott et al. 1981; Lapierre et al. 1984) and are typical for anxiety patients in general (cf. Lader 1975). With the exception of the effects on delta they can be interpreted as indicators of over-activation (Lapierre and Knott 1981; Lapierre et al. 1984). Interestingly, at baseline subsequent lactate panickers had greater sympathetic arousal (Liebowitz et al. 1985). The mechanism of the above changes is unclear since lactate, fluid volume, and the salt content of the solution may all have direct physiological effects not mediated through affective changes.

Griez and van den Hout (1983) reported that *inhalation of a 35% CO_2/65% oxygen mixture* led to rises in systolic blood pressure, cardiac output, and stroke volume. Diastolic blood pressure and pulse transit time decreased. Earlier studies had also found a drop in diastolic blood pressure, but no effects of CO_2 on systolic blood pressure (Ley and Walker 1973; Griez and van den Hout 1982; van den Hout and Griez 1982a, 1982b). Decreases in heart rate have been reported after single breath CO_2 inhalation (Ley and Walker 1973; Griez and van den Hout 1982). Other studies, however, found similar decreases after inhalation of air (van den Hout and Griez 1982a, 1982b). According to Griez and van den Hout (1983), heart rate decreases after CO_2 inhalation are an artifact of heart rate increases prior to the inhalation. Overall, the results of physiological measures are consistent with the notion that single inhalation of high CO_2 concentrations leads to higher activation in addition to peripheral vasodilatatory effects (Griez and van den Hout 1984) though heart rate and diastolic blood pressure may not follow this pattern.

Physiological effects of *prolonged inhalation of 5% CO_2* have recently been studied in our laboratory using the procedure of Gorman et al. (1984a). Consistent with elevated activation highly significant increases in heart rate as well as systolic and diastolic blood pressure were found (see below, Ehlers et al. in press a).

3.1.3. Biochemical Effects

In contrast to the results from physiological and self-report measures, *biochemical* effects of *lactate infusion* do not consistently indicate heightened arousal or stress-related changes in blood hormones (Bonn et al. 1971, 1973; Appleby et al. 1981; Gorman et al. 1984b; Liebowitz et al. 1985). The lack of consistent changes in peripheral catecholamines (Appleby et al. 1981; Liebowitz et al. 1985) might reflect the rather moderate levels of subjective anxiety reached with lactate. Similarly, the decreases in cortisol found by Liebowitz et al. (1985) argue against a powerful stressor-effect of lactate infusions. Many of the biochemical results reported may be direct effects of the infused lactate, such as hypocalcemia and mild metabolic alkalosis (Bonn et al. 1971, 1973; Liebowitz et al. 1985). Hypoglycemia was not observed (Gorman et al. 1984b). Although increases in bicarbonate and decreases in pCO_2 were more marked in panicking subjects than in nonpanicking subjects (Liebowitz et al. 1985), the changes were generally in the same direction in all subjects.

Griez and van den Hout (1984) found that *single inhalation of a 35% CO_2/65% oxygen* mixture immediately led to a severe respiratory alkolosis and rise in arterial pCO_2. After exhalation, a sharp drop in pCO_2 occurred followed by a hypocapnic overshoot. Report of symptoms coincided with the drop in arterial pCO_2. *Prolonged inhalation of 5% CO_2* in the protocol used by Gorman et al. (1984a) led to slight, not 'substantive', arterial acidosis, indicating a 'modest buildup' of CO_2.

3.2. Incidence of Lactate and CO_2-Induced Panic Attacks

Eight studies compared the responses of panic patients and normal control subjects to both lactate and placebo (Pitts and McClure 1967; Fink et al. 1971; Kelly et al. 1971; Bonn et al. 1971, 1973; Rifkin et al. 1981; Appleby et al. 1981; Liebowitz et al. 1984, 1985; Rainey et al. 1984a, 1984b; Freedman et al. 1984). Three other studies used clinical control populations (Lapierre et al. 1984; Gorman et al. 1985; Cowley et al., in press). The reported rates of *lactate-induced* panic in panic patients range from 26% (Lapierre et al. 1984) to 100% (Fink et al. 1971; Rifkin et al. 1981). Across all the above studies, 58% of the panic patients (158 of 271) panicked after roughly 12 minutes of lactate infusion. This compares to panic rates of 0% to 30% found for normal control subjects (across all studies 9%, or 7 of 76). Controls usually panicked after a longer period of time (3 to 6 more minutes, Kelly et al. 1971; Rainey et al. 1984b). Panic patients and normal controls differed not only in their response to lactate, but also in their response to *placebo* (panic rates of up to 36% for patients, consistently 0% for controls).

For patients with generalized anxiety disorder and with primary major depression and secondary panic attacks, panic rates similar to those of panic patients were reported (Lapierre et al. 1984; Cowley et al., in press). Patients with obsessive-compulsive neurosis showed lower rates (Gorman et al. 1985). Five other studies on panic patients that did not have control groups have not been included in the above analysis (Haslam 1974; Knott et al. 1981; Gorman et al. 1983, 1984b; Fyer et al. 1985). These studies reported panic rates in panic patients ranging from 64% to 100%.

Differences in the reported panic rates may be due to methodological differences. Interestingly, all studies yielding 100% panic rates in patients used samples of 10 or fewer patients. More recent studies tend to report lower panic rates. For example, the most recent study of the Columbia group (Gorman et al. 1985) found a panic rate of 54%. This compares to 72% reported by Liebowitz et al. (1984, 1985). Furthermore, the only double-blind study relying entirely on automatized (non-interactive) self-reports as criterion for panic attacks found a clearly lower proportion of attacks in patients than all other studies, namely 26% (Lapierre et al. 1984).

The only published study that compared the responses of panic patients and controls to CO_2 is the study of Gorman et al. (1984a) described above. 58% of their patients panicked (7 of 12) compared to none of only four controls. Our own replication of their study is described below (Ehlers et al. in press a).

3.3. Similarity of Laboratory-Induced and Naturally Occurring Panic

As we have specified elsewhere (Margraf et al. 1986), symptoms induced by lactate in panic patients and controls show considerable overlap with DSM-III criteria for panic attacks. Similarly, the two different protocols of *CO_2 inhalation* described above were found to produce DSM-III panic symptoms in panic patients (Gorman et al. 1984a) and normal volunteers (van den Hout and Griez 1984). The patients of Gorman et al. (1984a) reported that inhalation of 5% CO_2 resembled both the effects of lactate infusion and natural panic.

Rainey et al. (1984b) and Liebowitz et al. (1984) directly evaluated the similarity of individual symptom patterns during *lactate* and natural panic. Of 12 panic attacks induced by lactate in the study of Rainey et al., 3 were rated by the patient as somewhat or moderately similar to natural panic, 7 as very much so, and 2 as identical. Liebowitz et al. (1984) compared symptom patterns reported for lactate effects and natural panic attacks. Fear of dying, confusion, sense of unreality, difficulty with concentration, and sweating were more pronounced in natural panic. Lactate-induced attacks were accompanied by greater urinary urgency and twitching, which were interpreted as direct effects of the infused fluid volume and lactate-induced hypocalcemia.

Parallel to Maranon's (1924) finding that epinephrine injections resulted in so-called "cold" or "as if" emotions, Kelly et al. (1971) found that an unspecified number of patients during *lactate infusion* experienced only "the physiological concomitants of anxiety without the usual degree of mental fear" (p. 133). Similarly, Bonn et al. (1971, 1973) report that of 20 patients only 4 (20%) experienced overt panic, whereas 12 (60%) "would have panicked but for your presence, doctor".

It is difficult to judge the similarity between the physiological effects of lactate infusion or CO_2 inhalation and physiological concomitants of natural panic since the latter are largely unknown. Heart rate increases with lactate (on the average 21 bpm, Margraf et al. 1986) or CO_2 (Ehlers et al., in press a) seem to be lower than those recorded during natural panic by Lader and Mathews (1970) or Taylor et al. (1983, in press). On the other hand, a large percentage of panic attacks seem to occur without high heart rate elevations (Taylor et al., in press).

Overall, the question of similarity between effects of lactate or CO_2 and natural panic attacks remains open. While there are unquestionable similarities in symptoms and physiological changes, there are not enough direct and comprehensive investigations of this issue. Both subjective anxiety and heart rates accompanying lactate infusion or CO_2 inhalation are relatively moderate, and comparable data on naturally occurring panic attacks are lacking.

4. Panic Induction: Limitations and Open Questions

4.1. Methodological Considerations

Several important methodological criticisms apply to lactate infusion studies published so far (Margraf et al. 1986). Many studies fail to report essential information or report results incompletely and only qualitatively.

A critical factor limiting the interpretability of lactate infusion studies is that control strategies were generally inadequate. Most studies did not control sufficiently for demand characteristics and expectancy biases. Questionnaires did not contain bias control scales. Some studies even induced different expectations in their experimental groups by giving them different information before the infusion (e.g., Appleby et al. 1981). Furthermore, the subjects' blindness may have been endangered by different drip rates for placebo and lactate infusions and the presence of too many non-blind observers in studies using fixed order of infusions on a single day (Kelly et al. 1971; Knott et al. 1981; Appleby et al. 1981; Rifkin et al. 1981; Gorman et al. 1983, 1984b, 1985; Liebowitz et al. 1984, 1985; Rainey et al. 1984a, 1984b).

Most of these criticisms also apply to the CO_2 inhalation study of Gorman et al. (1984a), which had a pilot character (very few controls, sequence confound for CO_2 and hyperventilation). These authors did not design their study to assess the effects of CO_2. The series of studies on CO_2 inhalation presented by Griez and van den Hout (1984) was more carefully designed. However, this group did not directly compare panic patients and controls. Most of their non-treatment research was done in normal volunteers.

A general remaining problem is the methodology of determining whether or not a person had a panic attack during lactate infusion or CO_2 inhalation. There are no generally accepted objective criteria for panic attacks, and these attacks show considerable variation across and within individuals. Many studies on lactate infusion or CO_2 inhalation did not explicitly specify their criteria. This is especially relevant in single-blind studies where non-blind observers or the experimenters themselves determined whether or not panic attacks occurred.

A better approach to judge the effects of panic challenge tests would be to record multiple measures like symptoms, anxiety levels, physiological and biochemical changes and to compare their pattern with that of natural panic attacks. Interestingly, most studies did not even present data on subjective anxiety or use standard measures of anxiety, making it impossible to judge whether the 'intense apprehension, fear or terror' required by DSM-III (APA 1980) was induced. Psychophysiological and biochemical measures were rarely taken. Furthermore, most studies did not take the time-course of changes induced by lactate or CO_2 into consideration. Continuous or multi-point assessments were rarely used, although DSM-III clearly defines panic attacks as having a sudden onset and limited duration (p. 230–231).

4.2. Sensitivity and Specificity of Panic Challenges

The average sensitivity of 58% found for lactate infusion (see above) and CO_2 inhalation (Gorman et al. 1984a) is only moderate. With respect to specificity the results are even more problematic. The studies of Lapierre et al. (1984) and Cowley et al. (in press) did not find different panic rates for panic patients and patients with generalized anxiety disorder or major depression with secondary panic attacks. However, the Columbia group seems to find lower panic rates in patients with obsessive-compulsive disorder (Gorman et al. 1985) and social phobia (Liebowitz et al., in press, cited in Gorman et al. 1985).

It is also questionnable whether normal control subjects indeed show a qualitatively different response to lactate or CO_2, as is generally assumed. Significant qualitative differences would exist if core symptoms occurred exclusively in patients, or if clearly different patterns of symptoms were observed. However, lactate infusion studies reporting symptoms for both groups found similar response profiles which were characterized by paresthesias, tremor and shakiness, dizziness, palpitations, giddiness, dyspnea, and nervousness as well as increased autonomic arousal, hypocalcemia, and mild alkalosis. There appears to be no qualitative difference between the average patient and the average control for measures of anxiety and heart rate if baseline levels are taken into consideration (see below). Moreover, psychophysiological and biochemical changes occurred in most subjects regardless of diagnostic category and of observer determination of panic attacks.

Another important finding is that only panic patients, but not normal controls, "panic" in response to placebo. Insufficient control of expectancy biases and demand characteristics might contribute to this result. However, it is possible that we are dealing with a more general phenomenon in that panic patients might show more symptoms and physiological concomitants of anxiety than controls under a variety of stressful conditions. Thus, the basic idea of patients responding differently from controls, whether quantitatively or qualitatively, may be more true of the response to placebo or other stressors than the response to 'panic challenges'. A direct comparison of standard stress tests and CO_2 inhalation is presented later in this chapter (Ehlers et al., in press a).

4.3. Relevance of Baseline Levels of Anxiety and Arousal

It has consistently been found that panic patients reach higher levels of anxiety and physiological arousal than normal controls during lactate infusion. However, a closer look at the data reveals that the actual increase from baseline to lactate levels is similar for both groups. Panic patients as a group are more likely to panic, and as a group have higher baseline values than controls in anxiety (Kelly et al. 1971; Liebowitz et al. 1984, 1985; Rainey et al. 1984a, 1984b; Freedman et al. 1984), heart rate, systolic blood pressure and forearm blood flow (Kelly et al. 1971; Liebowitz et al. 1984, 1985), and have lower baseline levels of bicarbonate and pCO_2 (Bonn et al. 1971, 1973; Liebowitz et al. 1985). In addition, within the patient group, those with higher fearfulness, diastolic blood pressure, and heart rates at baseline are more likely to go on to panic during lactate infusion (Liebowitz et al. 1984, 1985).

That baseline state can influence the effects of arousing drugs has been reported as early as 1924. In a study of Maranon (1924), responses to epinephrine injection depended on whether the subject was calm or excited before the injection. Correspondingly, panic challenge tests may simply add to baseline arousal. More highly aroused subjects should in this case more likely be pushed across a tolerance threshold. In the next section, we present results from two of our own studies supporting this interpretation.

5. Two Studies on Panic Induction

The problems with previous panic induction studies outlined above led us to conduct our own studies. The first study investigated the role of baseline differences between panic patients and controls during lactate infusion (Ehlers et al., in press b). For this purpose, the time course of placebo and lactate-induced changes was monitored. We paid careful attention to the control of demand characteristics and expectancy biases. The experimenters' interaction with the subject was minimal during the infusion. In addition to the slow placebo infusion used in other studies, we introduced a second placebo condition in which normal saline was infused at a rate matching that of the lactate infusion.

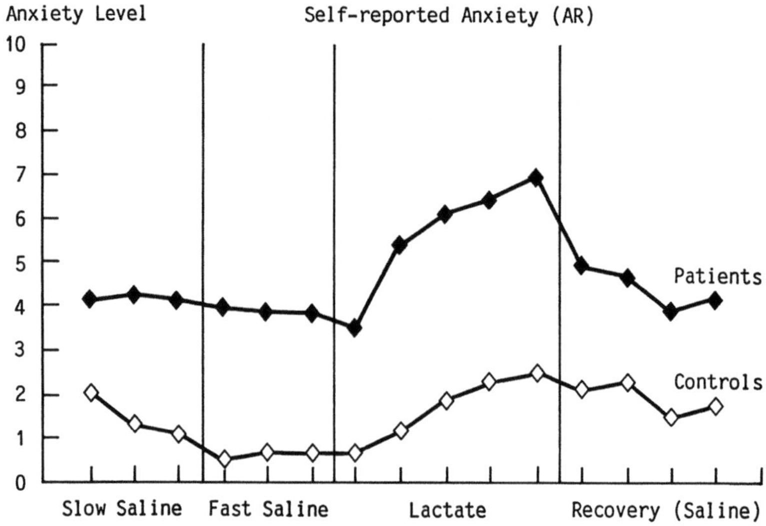

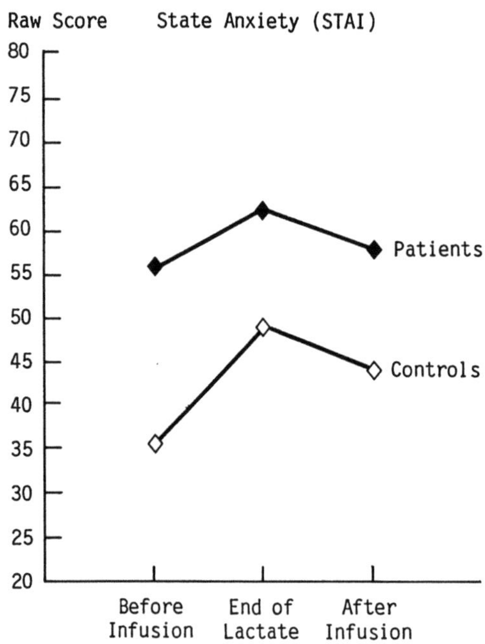

Fig. 1. Self-reported anxiety in panic patients and normal controls during infusions of saline (placebo) and sodium lactate (Ehlers et al., in press b). A single-blind procedure with a fixed sequence of infusions was used in this study. The Anxiety Rating Scale (AR) ranges from 0 (labelled "none") to 10 (labelled "extreme"). The AR was given every 5 min during the infusions. The state form of the State-Trait Anxiety Inventory (STAI, Spielberger et al. 1970) was given at the beginning of the session (before the infusions), at the end of the lactate infusion, and after the recovery period (saline). The results for heart rate were parallel to those for self-reported anxiety. Patients and controls only differed in their blood pressure response to lactate.

Ten female patients with panic disorder or agoraphobia with panic attacks and 10 female age-matched normal controls received infusions of normal saline (placebo) and sodium lactate in a single-blind design. Saline was infused slowly for 15 min. Then the infusion rate was increased to what would be used for the lactate infusion. After 15 min of fast saline infusion, 1.0 M racemic sodium lactate was infused at the rate of 15 mg/kg/hr for a maximum of 20 min. However, the lactate infusion was terminated before 20 min, if subjects reported severe anxiety or panic and asked to stop. The time course of changes in self-reported anxiety, heart rate and blood pressure was monitored.

Lactate increased anxiety (see Fig. 1) and cardiovascular arousal in both patients and controls. The changes appeared specific to

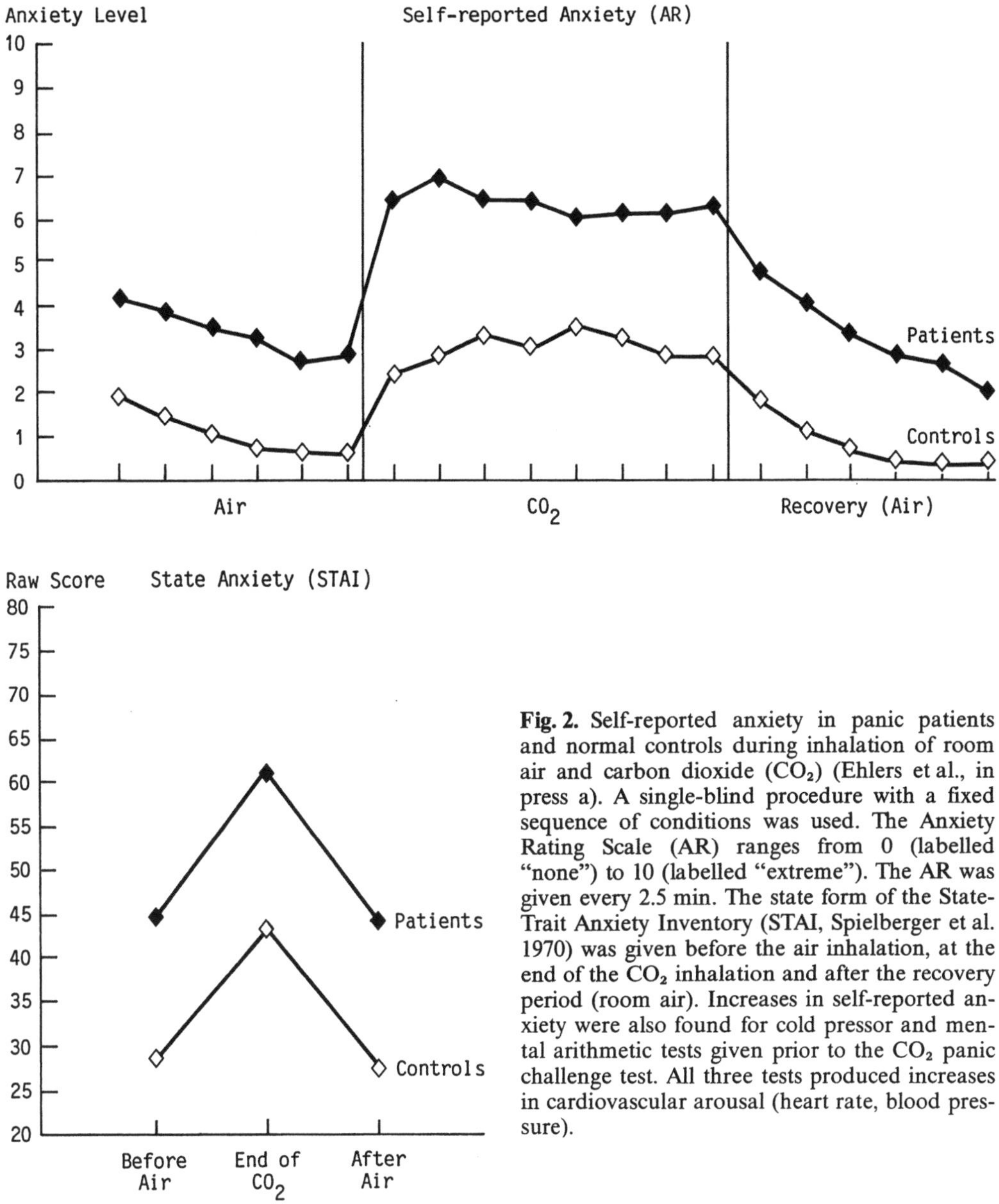

Fig. 2. Self-reported anxiety in panic patients and normal controls during inhalation of room air and carbon dioxide (CO_2) (Ehlers et al., in press a). A single-blind procedure with a fixed sequence of conditions was used. The Anxiety Rating Scale (AR) ranges from 0 (labelled "none") to 10 (labelled "extreme"). The AR was given every 2.5 min. The state form of the State-Trait Anxiety Inventory (STAI, Spielberger et al. 1970) was given before the air inhalation, at the end of the CO_2 inhalation and after the recovery period (room air). Increases in self-reported anxiety were also found for cold pressor and mental arithmetic tests given prior to the CO_2 panic challenge test. All three tests produced increases in cardiovascular arousal (heart rate, blood pressure).

lactate since they did not occur during the preceding saline infusion or on a previous test day without infusion. The most prominent difference between patients and controls was constantly elevated anxiety and heart rates in panic patients, beginning in the placebo period and continuing throughout the session. Lactate increased self-reported anxiety and heart rate equally in patients and controls. The only variables showing statistically different responses between patients and controls were systolic and diastolic blood pressure.

In four patients, the lactate infusion was stopped before 20 min had elapsed. These patients had higher anxiety levels than other patients and controls during the placebo infusion. Their heart rates increased at a faster rate with the lactate infusion, and showed larger decreases during the recovery period.

Symptom patterns described for lactate effects were quite similar to states of natural anxiety and panic. Patients, however, had a clear tendency to endorse somatic symptoms indiscriminately as measured by a response bias scale. Seven patients and seven controls rated the effects of lactate as similar to states of natural panic or extreme anxiety. A direct comparison of heart rates and anxiety ratings during lactate and during ambulatorily monitored panic attacks showed that lactate effects were of comparable magnitude to those of naturally occurring panic attacks.

The same pattern of results was replicated in our study (Ehlers et al., in press a) of CO_2 inhalation (see Fig. 2). We observed the time course of changes during CO_2 inhalation using the protocol of Gorman et al. (1984a). In addition, we addressed the question of specificity of this so-called panic induction method by comparing the effects of CO_2 with two standard stress tests, the cold pressor and mental arithmetic. Furthermore, we assessed the possible role of differential expectancies of patients and control subjects.

Subjects were 16 patients with panic disorder or agoraphobia with panic attacks and 18 age- and sex-matched normal controls. After a baseline, the cold pressor test and mental arithmetic were presented in balanced order. During the following CO_2 test, a concentration of 5.5% CO_2 was delivered through a gas mask for 20 min after subjects had breathed room air (placebo) for 15 min. The CO_2 inhalation was terminated before 20 min if subjects reported severe anxiety or panic and asked to stop. The time course of changes in self-reported anxiety, heart rate and blood pressure was closely monitored. To assess possible expectancy effects, responses to wearing the gas mask while breathing room air (1) prior to the CO_2 challenge and (2) on a previous occasion when no CO_2 was expected, were compared with the respective baselines.

Throughout the session, patients had higher anxiety and heart rate levels than controls. The effects of the standard stress tests and CO_2 were very similar. All three stressors led to highly significant increases in anxiety and cardiovascular arousal. The responses of panic patients and controls were similar. The only exception was that patients showed faster increases in heart rate and systolic blood pressure in response to CO_2. Three patients and one control asked to stop the CO_2 inhalation before 20 min had elapsed. These subjects had higher baseline levels of anxiety than subjects who completed the inhalation. The majority of subjects reported that the CO_2 inhalation was the most unpleasant test. 69% of the patients and 44% of the controls rated the effects of CO_2 as similar to usual panic attacks or extreme anxiety.

When subjects wore the gas mask without expecting CO_2, both groups showed similar increases in subjective anxiety compared to baseline, but no changes in cardiovascular arousal. In contrast, in anticipation of the panic challenge test, patients showed larger increases in cardiovascular arousal than control subjects.

The results of our two studies demonstrate that baseline differences have to be taken into account in the interpretation of 'panic induction' studies. They underline the crucial mediating role of expectancy effects.

6. Discussion and Conclusions

Results from lactate infusion and CO_2 inhalation studies have been interpreted as meaning that panic attacks are biologically distinct from other forms of anxiety. A review of the literature and our own studies demonstrate, however, that current evidence does not support a simple biological explanation of the anxiogenic effects of lactate and CO_2. Most studies have methodological flaws that severely limit the conclusions that can be drawn from them. The same limitations apply to other panic induction experiments using anxiety-inducing substances like caffeine, yohimbine, etc. (for a discussion, see Margraf et al. 1986).

In spite of these problems, certain facts have been established. First, baseline levels of anxiety and arousal are of paramount importance for the outcome of panic induction studies. Studies that have monitored the time course of changes before and during the panic challenge have consistently found that panic patients and control subjects differ in their baseline levels of anxiety and autonomic arousal as well as in the levels they reach under panic challenge conditions (Kelly et al. 1971; Liebowitz et al. 1984, 1985; Rainey et al. 1984a, 1984b; Freedman et al. 1984; Ehlers et al. in press a, in press b). In addition, patients who go on to panic are those who had higher baseline levels initially (Liebowitz et al. 1984, 1985; Ehlers et al., in press a, in press b).

A second fact that has emerged clearly is the limited sensitivity and specificity of lactate and CO_2 challenges. There are substantial proportions of panic patients that do not react significantly to either provocation. In addition, other stress tests such as the cold pressor test induce similar response patterns. Differences in the responses to different stressors are more a matter of degree than a matter of quality. The same applies to differences between the various patient groups and controls. Patients without panic disorder and even normal controls show response patterns similar to those of panic patients. Thus, current evidence does not indicate a specific action of lactate or CO_2 on patients prone to panic attacks. Consequently, response to these challenges cannot be regarded as a biological marker for a person's proneness to panic attacks, and these results do not provide support for the hypothesis that panic is a qualitatively different form of anxiety.

No definite conclusions can be drawn from the existing data about mechanisms underlying the anxiogenic effects of lactate and CO_2. As we have outlined elsewhere (Margraf et al. 1986), the proposed biological mechanisms do not sufficiently explain the results of lactate infusion studies. The contradictory interpretations proposed for the recent findings on CO_2 lend further support to this view. Based on their CO_2 studies and the effects of lactate infusion and hyperventilation (Lum 1981; Bonn et al. 1984; cf. the chapter by Margraf, Ehlers, Roth in this book), Griez and van den Hout (1984) conclude that "it appears that alkalisation of body fluids is a common denominator of natural and artificial panic" (p. 134). Prolonged inhalation of 5% or 5.5% CO_2 which also induces panic anxiety, however, results in mild acidosis (Gorman et al. 1984a). Similarly, interpretations focussing on central chemoreceptor sensitivity and an increase in cerebral CO_2 (Carr and Sheehan 1984; Liebowitz et al. 1985) are inconsistent with the finding of normal CO_2 chemoreceptor sensitivity in panic patients (Woods et al. 1985).

Any model explaining the results of panic induction studies must take cognitive and learning variables into account. This is emphasized by the placebo responsivity of panic patients (Rainey et al. 1984a, 1984b; Freedman et al. 1984), the patients' tendency to overreport somatic symptoms (Ehlers et al., in press b), some patients' reports of physiological symptoms without subjective anxiety (Kelly et al. 1971; Bonn et al. 1971, 1973), the anxiety-reducing effects of repeated lactate infusion or CO_2 inhalation or their combination (Bonn et al. 1971; Haslam 1974; Griez and van den Hout 1984), and the effects of different instructions (van den Hout and Griez 1982a). Even if panic patients and controls receive identical instructions, they are likely to have differential expectancies concerning the experimental procedure. This was demonstrated in the study by Ehlers et al. (in press a) where the patients' different expectations had a clear physiological impact. Furthermore, Guttmacher and Nelles (1984) recently presented the case of a patient who did not respond to lactate infusion after successful behavior therapy but had panicked prior to treatment. Together, these findings support the often postulated role of 'fear of fear' in panic and agoraphobic patients (Westphal 1871; Frankl 1975; Goldstein and Chambless 1978; Griez and van den Hout 1984; Beck and Emery 1985). For a more comprehensive description of psychophysiological models of panic see the chapter by Margraf, Ehlers, and Roth in this book.

7. References

Ackerman S, Sachar E (1974) The lactate theory of anxiety: A review and reevaluation. Psychosom Med 36:69–81

American Psychiatric Association (ed) (1980) Diagnostic and Statistical Manual of Mental Disorders, 3rd edn. American Psychiatric Press, Washington, D.C.

Appleby IL, Klein DF, Sachar E, Levitt M (1981) Biochemical indices of lactate-induced panic: A preliminary report. In: Klein DF, Rabkin J (eds) Anxiety: New research and changing concepts. Raven Press, New York

Beck AT, Emery GD (1985) Anxiety disorders and phobias. A cognitive perspective. Basic Books, New York

Bonn JA, Harrison J, Rees W (1971) Lactate-induced anxiety: Therapeutic application. Br J Psychiatry 119:468–470

Bonn JA, Harrison J, Rees W (1973) Lactate infusion in the treatment of "free-floating anxiety". Can Psychiatric Assoc J 18:41–45

Bonn JA, Redhead C, Timmons BA (1984) Enhanced adaptive behavioral response in agoraphobic patients pretreated with breathing retraining. Lancet 1984:665–669

Breggin PR (1964) The psychophysiology of anxiety. J Nerv Ment Dis 139:558–568

Carr DB, Sheehan DV (1984) Evidence that panic disorder has a metabolic cause. In: Ballenger JC (ed) Biology of agoraphobia. American Psychiatric Press, Washington, D.C.

Cowley DS, Dager SA, Dunner DL (in press) Lactate-induced panic in primary affective disorder

Ehlers A, Margraf J, Roth WT (in press a) Interaction of expectancy and physiological stressors in a laboratory model of panic. In: Hellhammer D, Florin I (eds) Neuronal control of bodily function – basic and clinical aspects. Vol. II. Psychological and biological approaches to the understanding of human disease. Martinus-Nijhoff, Boston

Ehlers A, Margraf J, Roth WT, Taylor CB, Maddock RJ, Sheikh J, Kopell MJ, McClenahan KL, Gossard D, Blowers GH, Agras WS, Kopell BS (in press b) Lactate infusions and panic attacks: Do patients and controls respond differently? Psychiatr Res

Elridge F (1968) Letter to the editor. N Engl J Med 278:629

Fink M, Taylor M, Volavka J (1971) Anxiety precipitated by lactate. N Engl J Med 281:1429

Foa EB, Steketee G, Young MC (1984) Agoraphobia: Phenomenological aspects, associated characteristics, and theoretical considerations. Clin Psychol Review 4:431–457

Frankl VE (1975) Paradoxical intention and dereflection. Psychotherapy 12:226–237

Freedman DX, Glass RM (1984) Psychiatry. JAMA 252:2223–2228

Freedman RR, Ianni P, Ettedgui E, Pohl R, Rainey JM (1984) Psychophysiological factors in panic disorder. Psychopathology 17 (Supplement 1):66–73

Freedman RR, Ianni P, Ettedgui E, Puthezhath N (1985) Ambulatory monitoring of panic disorder. Arch Gen Psychiatry 42:244–248

Fyer AJ, Liebowitz MR, Gorman JM, Davies SO, Klein DF (1985) Lactate vulnerability of remitted panic patients. Psychiatr Res 14:143–148

Goldstein AJ, Chambless DL (1978) A reanalysis of agoraphobia. Behavior Therapy 9:47–59

Gorman JM, Levy G, Liebowitz MR, McGrath P, Appleby IL, Dillon D, Davies SO, Klein DF (1983) Effect of acute beta adrenergic blockade on lactate-induced panic. Arch Gen Psychiatry 140:1079–1082

Gorman JM, Askanazi J, Liebowitz MR, Fyer AJ, Stein J, Kinney JM, Klein DF (1984a) Response to hyperventilation in a group of patients with panic disorder. Am J Psychiatry 141:857–861

Gorman JM, Martinez J, Liebowitz MR, Fyer AJ, Klein DF (1984b) Hypoglycemia and panic attacks. Am J Psychiatry 141:101–102

Gorman JM, Liebowitz MR, Fyer AJ, Dillon D, Davies SO, Stein J, Klein DF (1985) Lactate infusions in obsessive-compulsive disorder. Am J Psychiatry 142:864–866

Griez E, van den Hout MA (1982) Effects of carbondioxide-oxygen inhalations on subjective anxiety and some neurovegetative parameters. J Beh Ther Exp Psychiatry 13:27–32

Griez E, van den Hout MA (1983) Carbondioxide and anxiety. Cardiovascular effects of a single inhalation. J Beh Ther Exp Psychiatry 14:297–304

Griez E, van den Hout MA (1984) Carbondioxide and anxiety. Thesis, Rijksuniversiteit, Maastricht

Grosz H (1973) Lactate-induced anxiety: Hypothesis and experimental model. Br J Psychiatry 122:116–117

Grosz H, Farmer B (1969) Blood lactate in the development of anxiety symptoms. Arch Gen Psychiatry 21:611–619

Grosz H, Farmer B (1972) Pitts' and McClure's lactate-anxiety study revisited. Br J Psychiatry 120:415–418

Guttmacher LB, Nelles C (1984) In vivo desensitization of lactate-induced panic: A case study. Behavior Therapy 15:369–372

Hand I (1984) Verhaltenstherapie und Psychopharmaka bei Phobien? Welche Konsequenzen hat die „Entdeckung“ der Panic Disorder wirklich für die verhaltenstherapeutische Praxis und Forschung? In: Götze P (ed) Leitsymptom Angst. Springer, Berlin

Haslam M (1974) The relationship between the effect of lactate infusion on anxiety states and their amelioration by carbon dioxide inhalation. Br J Psychiatry 125:88–90

Henderson R (1968) Letter to the editor. N Engl J Med 278:629

Kelly D, Mitchell-Heggs N, Sherman D (1971) Anxiety and the effects of sodium lactate assessed clinically and physiologically. Br J Psychiatry 119:129–141

Klein DF (1981) Anxiety reconceptualized. In: Klein DF, Rabkin J (eds) Anxiety: New research and changing concepts. Raven Press, New York

Knott V, Chaudry R, Lapierre YD (1981) Panic induced by sodium lactate: Electrophysiological correlates. Prog Neuropsychopharmacology 5:511–514

Lader M (1975) The psychophysiology of mental illness. Routledge and Kegan Paul, London

Lader M, Mathews A (1970) Physiological changes during spontaneous panic attacks. J Psychosom Res 14:377–382

Lapierre YD, Knott VJ (1981) Psychophysiological correlates of mental disorders. In: Hrdina PD, Singhal RL (eds) Neuroendocrine regulation and altered behavior. Croom Helm, London

Lapierre YD, Knott VJ, Gray R (1984) Psychophysiological correlates of sodium lactate. Psychopharmacol Bull 20:50–57

Latimer P (1977) Carbondioxide as a reciprocal inhibitor in the treatment of neurosis. J Beh Ther Exp Psychiatry 8:83–85

Levitt EE (1972) A brief communication on the "psychiatric breakthrough" with emphasis on the hematology of anxiety. In: Spielberger CD (ed) Anxiety, vol. 1. Academic Press, New York

Ley R, Walker H (1973) Effects of carbondioxide-oxygen inhalation on heart rate, blood pressure and subjective anxiety. J Beh Ther Exp Psychiatry 4:223–228

Liebowitz MJ, Fyer AJ, Gorman JM, Dillon D, Appleby IL, Levy G, Anderson S, Levitt M, Palij M, Davies SO, Klein DF (1984) Lactate provocation of panic attacks: I. Clinical and behavioral findings. Arch Gen Psychiatry 41:764–770

Liebowitz MJ, Gorman JM, Fyer AJ, Levitt M, Dillon D, Levy G, Appleby IL, Anderson S, Palij M, Davies S, Klein DF (1985) Lactate provocation of panic attacks: II. Biochemical and physiological findings. Arch Gen Psychiatry 42:709–719

Lum LC (1981) Hyperventilation and anxiety state. J Royal Soc Med 74:1–4

Maranon G (1924) Contribution a l'étude de l'action emotive de l'adrenaline. Revue Fr Endocrinol 2:301–325

Margraf J, Ehlers A, Roth WT (1986) Sodium lactate infusions and panic attacks: A review and critique. Psychosom Med 48:23–51

Marks I (1983) Are there anticompulsive or antiphobic drugs? Review of evidence. Br J Psychiatry 143:338–347

Meduna LJ (ed) (1955) Carbon dioxide therapy. A neurophysiological treatment of nervous disorders. Charles Thomas, Springfield Illinois

Pitts F (1969) The biochemistry of anxiety. Sci Am 220:69–75

Pitts F, McClure J (1967) Lactate metabolism in anxiety neurosis. N Engl J Med 277:1329–1336

Rainey JM, Frohman CE, Freedman RR, Pohl RB, Ettedgui E, Williams M (1984a) Specificity of lactate infusion as a model of anxiety. Psychopharmacol Bull 20:45–49

Rainey JM, Pohl RB, Williams M, Knitter E, Freedman RR, Ettedgui E (1984b) A comparison of lactate and isoproterenol anxiety states. Psychopathology 17 (Supplement 1):74–82

Rifkin A, Klein DF, Dillon D, Levitt M (1981) Blockade by imipramine or desipramine of panic induced by sodium lactate. Am J Psychiatry 138:676–677

Shader R, Goodman M, Gever J (1982) Panic disorders: Current perspectives. J Clin Psychopharmacol 2 (Supplement):2S–10S

Sheehan D (1982) Panic attacks and phobias. N Engl J Med 307:156–158

Slater SL, Levy A (1966) The effects of inhaling a 35% CO_2/65% O_2 mixture upon anxiety in neurotic patients. Beh Res Ther 4:309–316

Spielberger CD, Gorsuch RL, Lushene RE (1970) STAI Manual. Consulting Psychologist's Press. Palo Alto, California

Taylor CB, Telch MJ, Havvik D (1983) Ambulatory heart rate changes during panic attacks. J Psychiatr Res 17:261–266

Taylor CB, Sheikh J, Agras WS, Roth WT, Margraf J, Ehlers A, Maddock RJ, Gossard D (in press) Ambulatory heart rate changes in panic attack patients. Am J Psychiatry

van den Hout M, Griez E (1982a) Cognitive factors in carbon dioxide therapy. J Psychosom Res 26:209–214

van den Hout M, Griez E (1982b) Cardiovascular and subjective responses to inhalation of carbondioxide. Psychother Psychosom 37:75–82 van den Hout MA, Griez E (1984) Panic symptoms after inhalation of carbondioxide. Br J Psychiatry 144:503–507

Westphal C (1871) Die Agoraphobie, eine neuropathische Erscheinung. Archiv für Psychiatrie und Nervenkrankheiten 3:138–161

Woods SW, Charney DS, Loke J, Goodman WK, Redmond E, Henninger GR (1985) CO_2 chemoreceptor sensitivity in panic patients. Paper presented at the 138th Annual Meeting of the American Psychiatric Association, Dallas, Texas

Wolpe J (1958) Psychotherapy by reciprocal inhibition. Stanford University Press, Stanford, California

7. Agoraphobia and the Hyperventilation Syndrome – the Role of Interpretations of Complaints

Bert Garssen

1. Introduction

Agoraphobia is considered by many authors to be a secondary reaction to the occurrence of panic attacks (Roberts 1964; Mendel and Klein 1969; Grunhaus et al. 1981). Such a causal relation is plausible. It has been demonstrated, that the majority (69 to 100%) of agoraphobic patients have panic attacks (Roberts 1964; DiNardo et al. 1983; Marks et al. 1983; Torgesen 1983; Garvey and Tuason 1984; Thyer et al. 1985). The first panic attacks occurred before, or at least at the same time as the onset of the agoraphobic complaints (Roberts 1964; Garvey and Tuason 1984).

Patients often describe the first attacks as unexpected. Suddenly there was the pounding of the heart, the feeling of breathlessness, the shivering and unsteadiness; it was like losing control or fainting and one was struck by the fear of a terrible thing happening. Doctors being consulted thereafter could not find a definite cause. However, the person's doubt was not set at rest by the doctor's reassurance that it was simply "nervous overstrain". Suspicion was fed by the frequent reoccurrence of complaints, and then the constant, anxious anticipation of new attacks set in. Thereafter, specific "agoraphobic" situations are avoided, such as being alone, being in crowded situations, or situations difficult to escape from in case of an impending attack (buses, trains, lifts, sitting in the middle of a row).

We have studied the relationship between the Hyperventilation Syndrome (HVS) and agoraphobia. There is a striking similarity between the description of panic attacks in the DSM-III and the description of the Hyperventilation Syndrome (Weimann 1968; Lum 1976; Magarian 1982; Brashear 1983; Garssen and Rijken 1986). So, what applies to panic attacks and its relation to agoraphobia should also hold for the HVS. It appeared from our study that 61% of the agoraphobic patients also fulfilled the criteria for the HVS (Garssen et al. 1983).

There is no simple cause–effect relationship between the occurrence of hyperventilation attacks (or panic attacks in general) and agoraphobia, which follows from the mere fact that panic disorder does not always lead to agoraphobic complaints. In the first place more factors are involved than fear of new attacks. Judging from the answers to a questionnaire and a structured interview, social anxiety and avoidance seemed to play an additional role and were the most important factors in a few patients (Garssen et al. 1983). In the second place, the occurrence of attacks of bodily symptoms are not in themselves decisive; it is the way attacks are interpreted and coped with.

Probably, periods of tightness in the chest, heart sensations, dizziness, unsteadiness and tension will now and then occur in many healthy subjects, who never develop HVS, panic disorder, or agoraphobia. We would suggest that those persons generally interprete their complaints in a sober way, something like: "When I think about it, these complaints do not come quite unexpectedly. There were many emotional problems that burdened me these past weeks. Symptoms would occur sooner or later." Given this interpretation, the person probably will choose a coping strategy that is effective for him. An adequate coping behaviour may be to distance oneself from work or emotional problems, and to look for advice or help to solve these problems. Complaints will then gradually disappear and probably not reappear.

However, many people will not be capable of such a down-to-earth interpretation. For them the complaints came unexpectedly. Complaints may afterwards be (incorrectly) ascribed to somatic illnesses, such as cancer or a heart disease. If the first attack was an elusive phenomenon to the subject, or was attributed to an anxiety-inducing cause, anxious anticipation of new attacks will develop. This will lead to a high level of physiological arousal, which increases the chance of new attacks occurring and thereby also increases the chance of developing agoraphobic avoidance behavior.

Complaints may also be attributed to stressful situations that occurred in the preceeding weeks or months, or to the actual situation in which the attack occurred. Take for instance a person who has longstanding quarrels with his parents in law, living with him. On his way to a party he experiences complaints such as palpitations, tightness in the chest, and dizziness. The person may see these complaints as induced by the stressful events (=the quarrels) that had gone before. This attribution is probably correct. It is in line with current views about the etiological factors in the HVS, though a scientific explanation would mention in addition a specific psychophysiological mechanism to explain the deviant respiratory behaviour (Garssen 1980). So, it may be said that the person had some insight and used a rather sober explanation for his complaints. We predict that such insight will probably not lead to anxious anticipation and will not result in a serious illness condition. On the other hand, the person may ascribe his complaints to the actual situation (=going to the party). Then he must conclude that he cannot manage such situations. This insecurity will generalize to other situations and to anxious anticipation.

In the present study we investigated the role of interpretations in HVS patients. It was predicted that a more serious illness condition would develop, 1) the more the first attacks were seen as elusive, 2) the more complaints were attributed to a severe, somatic illness, 3) the more they were ascribed to the actual situation and 4) the less they were seen as induced by stressful situations in the weeks or months before the first attacks.

This paper reports the results of the first series of eleven patients.

2. Methods

Outpatients from the psychiatric clinic were selected on basis of their answers to a short "HVS-questionnaire" (van Doorn et al. 1983). Patients suspected to be HVS patients were invited for a first session.

In this session they were asked to fill in the "extensive Questionnaire of Somatic Complaints" (exQSC). The exQSC (Garssen et al. 1983) asked with respect to 33 complaints how often they had occurred in the last month. Most of the symptoms mentioned by Weimann (1968, p. 4) were included. In the diagnosis and the data-evaluation only complaints that occurred at least once a week were considered. In the subsequent anamnestic interview patients were – among other things – asked when their attacks had begun. At the end of the session the hyperventilation provocation test was done. Patients were urged to breath as deeply and rapidly as possible for 1½ minutes. The alveolar carbon dioxide pressure had to decrease to at least 20 mm Hg. The patient was diagnosed as a HVS patient, if the complaints during this test were recognized as similar to the symptoms during spontaneous attacks. Only patients, who were diagnosed as HVS patients and could clearly remember their first attack, were invited for the second session.

The most difficult part of the study was to get reliable answers to questions about interpretations of complaints when they first occurred. For that end patients were first brought to imagine as clearly and lively as possible the details of the day of the first attack. Imagination was guided by questions like: "Please, return now to the day of your first attack you mentioned in the first session ... what day of the week is it? ... is it in the morning/afternoon/evening? ... are you at home? ... In what room? ... Are you alone? ... What are you doing? ... Do you already feel complaints? ... What kind of complaints? ..." and so on. Imagination was started after a period of relaxation and was done with the eyes closed. The events of the day passed chronologically and were discussed as happening in the present. Next questions were put in terms like: 1. "When you are thinking about what happened this day, do you have any idea why the complaints have come?". In the same way was asked if the patient thought 2) complaints had come because of a somatic illness, such as heart disease, cancer or brain disease, 3) complaints had been induced by circumstances occurring that day, such as being in a shop or going to a party, 4) complaints had come because of stressful events in the preceeding weeks or months.

Sessions were run by two investigators; one in turn was the interviewer, or was only listening and observing. After the second session the two investigators scored the opinions of the patients with respect to the four questions. Four point scales were used. A score of one was given when the patient had no idea about what caused his complaints (question 1), and when the patient absolutely did not think his complaints were induced by somatic illnesses (question 2), the actual situation (question 3), or stressful situations in the preceeding weeks or months (question 4). A score of four was given if the patient had definite, positive opinions with respect to the four questions.

The imagination period was tape recorded. An independent judge listened to these tapes and rated in the same way the opinions of the patient. Most ratings differed only slightly (=one point) and then the judgement of the independent rater was decisive. Ratings that differed more than one point only occurred in 7% of the (11×4) questions that were put. If so, the tape was replayed and a common opinion was formulated.

Then the opinion scores of the patients were related to the seriousness of their current somatic and phobic complaints. The total number of complaints, as scored to the exQSC, was taken as a measure of the seriousness of somatic complaints. The anxiety level was determined with the State Trait Anxiety Inventory (STAI) of Spielberger. Phobic complaints were scored on the Fear Survey Schedule (FSS) of Wolpe and Lang. The total FSS-score was used, as were the sumscores to the social phobia and agoraphobia subscales.

Spearman Rank Correlation Coefficients were calculated. Significance level was at $p=0.05$ for a two-tailed test.

3. Results

Correlation coefficients are given in Table 1. Results will be discussed per item:

Item 1. It appeared that the less causes for complaints were known to the patients – that is, the lower they scored on the first item – the higher was the number of somatic complaints. See the negative, though not significant correlation of 0.57. However, correlations with the anxiety and phobia scores were low.

Item 2. Positive correlations were expected for the second question. It was predicted, that the more patients had ascribed their complaints to a serious illness, the higher would be the number of complaints. However, correlations were negative.

Table 1. The Relation Between Interpretations of Complaints and Somatic and Phobic complaints

	QSC	TRA	STA	FSS	FSS1 (social phobia)	FSS2 (agora-phobia)
1. "Any idea about the causes of the complaints?"	−0.57	−0.28	−0.36	−0.06	0.07	−0.28
2. "Caused by somatic illnesses?"	−0.21	−0.50	−0.52	−0.26	−0.05	−0.52
3. "Induced by the actual situation?"	0.18	0.15	0.39	0.39	0.30	0.67*
4. "The consequence of stressful situations in the past?"	−0.76**	−0.19	−0.27	−0.18	−0.15	−0.34

* $0.01 < p \leq 0.05$; ** $p \leq 0.01$

QSC = Questionnaire of Somatic Complaints N=11
TRA = Trait Anxiety
STA = State Anxiety
FSS = Fear Survey Schedule

Item 3. It appeared that the more patients thought their complaints were induced by the actual situation (circumstances on the day of the first attack), the higher their phobic scores were. See the positive correlations to the FSS-total and subscores, especially the significant correlation with the agoraphobia subscale. The correlation with the somatic complaints scores were low.

Item 4. It appeared that the less complaints were ascribed to stressful situations in the past, the higher the number of somatic complaints. See the significant correlation coefficient of −0.76. The correlations with phobiascores were also negative – as was predicted – but low.

4. Discussion

It is generally assumed that the interpretation of attacks as coming unexpectedly – leading to a feeling of loss of control and to anxiety – contributes to the development of secondary avoidance behaviour. However, the role of interpretations has never been directly studied. Changing cognitions about bodily complaints has been used as part of therapeutic approaches. For instance, Clark et al. (1985) describe one element of their "respiratory control" procedure as "explanation of the effects of overbreathing, and reattribution of the cause of a patient's attack to hyperventilation". To strengthen their instructions they let the patient hyperventilate voluntarily. A third element was training in a respiratory control technique. Their approach led to a reduction in number of panic attacks and in phobic anxiety. However, because their treatment procedure consisted of several elements, the effect of changing interpretations cannot be properly evaluated. There are no other studies that investigated explicitly the role of cognitions about somatic complaints in patients with agoraphobia and/or panic attacks.

In the present study the variation in interpretations within the group of HVS patients was related to the seriousness of their current illness condition. We tried to find out what patients thought about their complaints when they occurred for the first time. One might dispute if people can remember in sufficient detail opinions they had months ago. However, for most patients the event was of vital interest. To stimulate recollection, patients were led to imagine relevant details of that particular day, before asking what they thought at that time about their complaints. For this study only patients were selected who could remember the onset of their attacks. Patients gave quite vivid descriptions of the day in question. Afterwards they were asked if events were remembered as occurring in the present. All but one patient – who was skipped – said, they could. So, one may accept with some certainty the trueness of the patient's statements.

Most of the correlations appeared to be in the predicted direction, though only some were significant. To our surprise one prediction – an assumption that is often made and seems self-evident – was not confirmed, namely the prediction that attributing one's complaints to a severe illness would lead to anxious anticipation and so to a more serious illness condition. The discussion of this unexpected finding can be better delayed till more data are gathered.

The predicted correlations were derived from a model that assumes a cause–effect relation between certain interpretations of complaints and the current illness state. For instance, it was supposed that attributing one's complaints to stressful situations occurring in the weeks or months before the attack, would promote adequate coping and so would contribute to a favorable illness condition. Of course, our data do not prove such a causal relationship, but they are at least in line with the model.

5. References

Brashear RE (1983) Hyperventilation Syndrome. Lung 161:257–273

Clark DM, Salkovskis PM, Chalkley AJ (1985) Respiratory control as a treatment for panic attacks. J Beh Ther Eyp Psychiat 16:23–30

DiNardo PA, O'Brien GT, Barlow DH, Waddell MT, Blanchard EB (1983) Reliability of DSM-III anxiety categories using a new structured interview. Arch Gen Psychiatry 40:1070–1074

Doorn P van, Colla P, Folgering H (1983) Een vragenlijst voor hyperventilatieklachten. De Psycholoog 18:573–577

Garssen B (1980) Role of stress in the development of the Hyperventilation Syndrome. Psychother Psychosomat 33:214–225

Garssen B, Veenendaal W van, Bloemink R (1983) Agoraphobia and the Hyperventilation Syndrome. Beh Res Ther 21:643–649

Garssen B, Rijken H (1986) Clinical aspects and treatment of the Hyperventilation Syndrome. To be published in: Beh Psychother 14

Garvey MJ, Tuason VB (1984) The relationship of panic disorder to Agoraphobia. Comprehens Psychiat 25:529–531

Grunhaus L, Glocer S, Weisstub E (1981) Panic attacks: A review of treatment and pathogenesis. J Nerv Ment Dis 169:608–613

Lum LC (1976) The syndrome of habitual chronic hyperventilation. In: OW Hill (ed) Modern trends in Psychosomatic Medicine 3. Butterworths, London pp 196–230

Magarian GJ (1982) Hyperventilation Syndromes: infrequently recognized common expressions of anxiety and stress. Medicine 61:219–236

Mendel JGC, Klein DF (1969) Anxiety attacks with subsequent agoraphobia. Comprehens Psychiat 10:190–195

Marks IM, Gray S, Cohen D, Hill R, Manson D, Ramm E, Stern R (1983) Imipramine and brief therapist-aided exposure in agoraphobics having self-exposure homework. Arch Gen Psychiatry 40:153–162

Roberts AH (1964) Housebound housewives – A follow-up study of a phobic anxiety state. Brit J Psychiat 110:191–197

Thyer BA, Himle J, Curtis GC, Cameron OG, Nesse RM (1985) A comparison of panic disorder and agoraphobia with panic attacks. Comprehens Psychiat 26:208–214

Torgesen S (1983) Genetic factors in anxiety disorders. Arch Gen Psychiatry 40:1085–1089

Weimann G (1968) Das Hyperventilationssyndrom. Urban & Schwarzenberg, München

8. Panic Disorder – Overlap with Symptoms of Somatization Disorder

Roy King, Jürgen Margraf, Anke Ehlers, and Richard Maddock

1. Introduction

Panic disorder shows a highly characteristic profile of symptoms that can be described on several different levels. These include the behavioral – the phobic avoidance of certain external situations of chronic patients, or the active, help-seeking behavior of acutely anxious patients; the emotional – the prototypic 'intense apprehension, fear or terror' of the acute attack; and the somatic – a multitude of autonomic and somatic symptoms. It is the latter feature that usually distinguishes best between panic disorder patients and patients with generalized anxiety disorder (Hoehn-Saric 1981, 1982; Anderson et al. 1984). The behavioral aspects of panic disorder and agoraphobia have been well investigated (Mathews et al. 1981; Thorpe and Burns 1983) and a number of studies of the cognitive and emotional aspects have recently been undertaken (Butler and Mathews 1983; Hibbert 1984; Mathews and MacLeod 1985). The somatic complaints that are central to most patients' experience of panic (Katon 1984), however, have only been superficially studied. It is this visceral aspect of panic disorder that we wish to explore in this work.

Typically, somatic symptoms of panic have been ascribed to a rather loosely defined sympathetic activation during states of intense anxiety. Alternatively, Tyrer (1973, 1976) has hypothesized that patients with predominantly 'somatic' anxiety as opposed to 'psychic' anxiety show a more accurate perception of bodily processes. This could make them more sensitive to changes in these functions. In a pilot study of anxious patients with heterogeneous diagnoses, Tyrer et al. (1980) found that patients with somatic anxiety showed indeed significantly more accurate cardiac awareness than anxious patients with predominantly psychic anxiety.

The recent epidemiological catchment area studies of the prevalence of psychiatric disorders in the United States indicate an odds ratio of 97 (Boyd et al. 1984), reflecting an association between somatization

Acknowledgments: This work was supported by grants from the Robert Wood Johnson and MacArthur Foundations. We wish to thank Alicia Fritchle for her help in preparing the manuscript.

and panic in the general population. There may be significant overlap between individuals who satisfy the criteria for somatization disorder and those who satisfy criteria for panic disorder. Since agoraphobic patients in general are more severely disabled than simple panic disorder patients, a relationship between somatization and phobic avoidance could be expected.

In this paper we will report the results of a pilot study that specifically tested the hypothesis that individuals with panic disorder satisfy the criteria for somatization disorder and that somatization is associated with significant phobic avoidance in patients with panic disorder and agoraphobia with panic attacks. In addition, we tested the hypothesis that individuals with multiple somatic complaints have an increased self-reported visceral sensitivity. Finally, since somatization has been conceived of as a trait rather than a state variable, we tested the stability over time of self-reported multiple somatic complaints.

2. Methods

2.1. Subjects

Our patient population consisted of 44 females who met DSM-III (APA 1980) criteria for panic disorder or agoraphobia with panic attacks as established by a structured clinical interview (SCID-UP, Spitzer and Williams 1984). The SCID-UP includes both a symptom cut-off (at least four symptoms out of a specified list) and a temporal cut-off (majority of symptoms start within 10 minutes) for panic attacks. Patients with a history of major depressive episodes were excluded if the onset of panic disorder was not clearly separated temporally from the depressive episodes. The distribution of ages (mean ± SD) for the panic patients was 35.4 ± 10.2 and for controls was 37.2 ± 11.0. Furthermore, the duration of panic disorder for the patient population was 3.9 ± 2.7 years. The control group consisted of 27 nonanxious females that were carefully screened for the absence of any history of psychiatric problems. The structured interviews were conducted by clinicians with special training and experience with the SCID-UP. All subjects were in good physical health as determined by history and physical examination.

2.2. The Self-Report Inventory for Somatic Symptoms (SISS)

We developed a self-report questionnaire to measure somatization, visceral sensitivity, and nonspecific neurotic symptoms. The somatization subscale (TSDS for 'total somatization disorder score') consists of a symptom checklist containing the 37 physical symptoms that make up the DSM-III diagnosis of somatization disorder. Subjects were asked whether they had experienced any of these symptoms to such a degree that it caused him or her to see a physician, alter his or her life pattern, or to take medicine other than aspirin. Furthermore, these symptoms were not explained by some diagnosable physical disorder or drug intake. A second subscale (PSYCH) consists of a checklist of nonspecific neurotic symptoms that include anxiety, fatigue, hopeless feelings, suicidal feelings or acts, and angry spells. The scores on the TSDS and PSYCH subscales are the number of symptoms endorsed. Visceral sensitivity was measured by two Lickert scales ranging from 1 to 7. The first scale asked whether the individual was particularly aware of or sensitive to cardiovascular perceptions such as palpitations. The second scale asked the same question for gastrointestinal sensations such as abdominal bloating cramps. These scales were denoted 'cardiovascular awareness' (CVA) and 'gastrointestinal awareness' (GIA).

2.3. Procedure

The SISS was given to patients before they participated in different treatment studies conducted by the Laboratory for the Study of Behavioral Medicine and the Laboratory for Clinical Psychopharmacology and Psychophysiology at Stanford University and the Palo Alto Veterans Administration

Medical Center. In addition to the SISS, a subgroup of 27 subjects completed a Beck Depression Inventory (Beck and Beck 1972). Mobility Inventory (Chambless et al. 1985), Beck's Sociotropy scale (Beck et al. 1983), and the state form of the State-Trait Anxiety Inventory (STAI/S, Spielberger et al. 1970) at their first visit to the laboratory. All subjects were required to be drug-free at the time of testing and benzodiazepine screens were performed to test compliance with these instructions. Informed consent was obtained from all subjects prior to participation.

3. Results

3.1. Psychometric Properties of the SISS

Both the TSDS and PSYCH subscales of the SISS demonstrated good internal consistency. Cronbach alpha scores were 0.88 for TSDS and 0.76 for PSYCH. Item intercorrelations and item-total correlations were high. Retest reliability was obtained by giving the SISS a second time six weeks after the initial testing. All SISS subscales showed good retest reliability with coefficients of 0.78 for TSDS, 0.84 for PSYCH, 0.72 for gastrointestinal awareness, and 0.95 for cardiovascular awareness.

3.2. Differences between Panic and Control Groups

Table 1 shows the results for the comparison of the panic and control groups by means of t-tests for the SISS subscales.

The panic group clearly was higher in the self-report of somatization symptoms, nonspecific neurotic symptoms, gastrointestinal awareness, and cardiovascular awareness. It is interesting to note that 12 out of the 44 panic patients reported more than 14 symptoms, the cut-off defined by DSM-III criteria for somatization disorder. In the control group, no subject reported more than 14 symptoms. This difference was highly significant in a chi-square test with Yates correction (chi-square $=7.0$, $p<0.005$, df $=1$).

3.3. Relationship with Phobic Avoidance and Major Depression

To investigate the relationship of somatization with clinical depression and phobic avoidance, we performed two-way ANOVA's with the SCID-UP diagnoses of a history of major depressive episodes (present, absent) and of significant phobic avoidance (no phobic avoidance, limited phobic avoidance, extensive phobic avoidance) as factors. The results showed that a history of major depressive episodes was not significantly associated with TSDS [$F(1,36)=3.22$, $p<0.08$]. However, confirming our hypothesis, the level of phobic avoidance was highly significantly associated with TSDS [$F(2,35)=9.64$, $p<0.0004$]. There was no significant interaction effect [$F(2,36)=1.04$]. The mean TSDS score for patients with extensive phobic avoidance (agoraphobia) was 16.1 as opposed to 9.0 for panic disorder without avoidance and 7.1 for limited phobic avoidance. Thus, the patients with agoraphobia showed the most pronounced increment in somatization disorder-like symptomatology.

3.4. Relationships with Other Measures

Table 2 shows the correlation of TSDS with other scales and variables.

Consistent with the comparison of the different diagnostic subgroups reported above, there was a significant correlation between phobic avoidance as measured by the mobility alone score of the Mobility Inventory and the TSDS score. As predicted by our hypotheses, both gastrointestinal and cardiovascular awareness correlated highly with somatization. In addition, somatization correlated with Beck's sociotropy scale which is a measure of social dependence and with nonspecific neurotic symptoms as measured by the PSYCH subscale of the SISS. It is important to note that there was no correlation between TSDS and either age or duration of panic disorder. A second important finding is that TSDS was independent of state anxiety as

Table 1. Self-report Inventory for Somatic Symptoms (SISS): Differences between panic patients and controls

Subscale	TSDS Total somatization disorder score	PSYCH Nonspecific neurotic symptoms	GIA Gastrointestinal awareness	CVA Cardiovascular awareness
Patients	9.1 (±5.4)	2.5 (±1.5)	5.2 (±2.0)	5.7 (±1.5)
Controls	2.1 (±2.5)	0.6 (±1.2)	2.5 (±1.6)	2.2 (±1.5)
t-test	p<0.0001	p<0.0001	p<0.0001	p<0.0001

Means (± standard deviations) are presented for the subscales of the SISS

Table 2. Correlations of TSDS (Total Somatization Disorder Score) with other scales and variables

Variable	Pearson correlation	Level of significance
Age	0.20	ns
Duration of panic disorder	0.12	ns
State anxiety (STAI/S, Spielberger et al. 1970)	0.09	ns
Sociotropy (Beck et al. 1983)	0.53	p<0.01
Mobility when accompanied (Chambless et al. 1985)	0.32	ns
Mobility when alone (Chambless et al. 1985)	0.46	p<0.02
Beck depression inventory (Beck and Beck 1972)	0.59	p<0.002
PSYCH (Nonspecific neurotic symptoms)	0.78	p<0.0001
CVA (Cardiovascular awareness)	0.43	p<0.005
GIA (Gastrointestinal awareness)	0.49	p<0.001

measured by the STAI/S at the first laboratory visit. Thus, anxiety in a new situation was unrelated to somatization symptoms even though panic patients have much higher state anxiety than the controls at this visit.

4. Discussion

In a controlled study of panic disorder and agoraphobia with panic attacks we found the hypothesized significant overlap between the somatization and panic syndromes. Not only had panic patients higher average somatization scores than normal controls, but over a quarter of them also qualified for a DSM-III diagnosis of somatization disorder. Somatization was furthermore significantly correlated with reported visceral sensitivity and with measures of phobic avoidance and social dependence, but not with state anxiety. Finally, somatization showed at least short-term stability over time.

Panic disorder seems to be characterized by both high state anxiety and high somatization. These two factors appear to be independent of each other. This is in contradiction to the notion that high somatization could simply represent a consequence of a long history of panic attacks. Furthermore, if high somatization was due to such a sensitization process, one would expect to see significant correlations with duration of panic disorder and maybe age. However, this is clearly not the case in our sample. It is thus conceivable that panic disorder is the result of the interaction of at least these two processes, namely heightened state anxiety and a heightened tendency to somatisize. The relationship of both social dependence (sociotropy) and phobic avoidance (mobility when alone) with somatization may indicate that those individuals with the highest level of somatization find their phobic symptoms to be most intense when they are alone rather than with an important significant other. Alternatively, possible consequences of symptoms could be appraised as more dangerous without the potential help of others.

Possible neurophysiological substrates for the mechanisms underlying state anxiety and somatization are suggested by recent neurobiological and neuropsychological studies. Gray (1982) has proposed a highly developed and well researched model for anxiety processes that involves the frontal cortex and septo-hippocampal systems enhancing a cognitive "checking" process for novel or aversive stimuli. A possible substrate for the mechanisms influencing somatization can be inferred from studies attempting to delineate the cortical, subcortical, and brain stem circuits involved in visceral perception. Animal studies implicate the amygdala as a central station in the processing of visceral emotional information. In rodents, amygdaloid lesions can reduce aggressiveness, conditioned emotional reactions, both active and passive responses to frustration, and conditioned taste aversion (Sarter and Markowitsch 1985; Cormier 1981). In primates, the same lesions can reduce social attachment behavior. Stimulation, on the other hand, can cause enhanced cardiovascular, gastrointestinal, and respiratory autonomic activity. Other work on primates has indicated that the presence of others during avoidance conditioning can reduce the adreno-cortical response to aversive stimuli (Stanton et al. 1985). In addition, the central and peripheral release of neuropeptide hormones, such as vasopressin arginine, can enhance avoidance learning by presumably changing memory or attentional processes (Koob et al. 1985). During states of heightened anxiety, all individuals may undergo the release of large quantities of vasopressin or other hormones and neurotransmitters.

These findings are consistent with the features of panic and somatization discussed in this chapter. They are also consistent with the observed relationship between somatization and social dependence. In susceptible individuals, releases of neuropeptides such as vasopressin could lead to increased functional activity in the parts of the amygdala that are central to the processing of visceral information. These events could function as internally generated triggers for seemingly spontaneous and unpredictable panic attacks (Margraf et al. 1986). They could also act as aversive cues that enhance the process of learning to avoid the external stimuli that are concurrent with these periods of heightened anxiety.

Finally, it is interesting to note that the original studies on somatization disorder conducted by Guze et al. (1967) diagnosed hysteria (somatization disorder) even in the presence of anxiety neurosis. Thus, the early work on the familial transmission of somatization disorder is probably confounded with panic disorder.

The factors underlying the relationship between panic attacks and somatization need to be investigated more directly in future studies. The various hypotheses outlined in this chapter could be tested by studying individuals with somatization disorder without any panic attacks and with generalized anxiety disorder. The effects of various treatments of panic disorder on subjects with high somatization could give us valuable information. Finally, it seems worthwhile to pursue the neuroanatomical and neurophysiological mechanisms discussed here.

5. References

Anderson DJ, Noyes R, Crowe RR (1984) A comparison of panic disorder and generalized anxiety disorder. Am J Psychiatry 141:572–575

American Psychiatric Association, Committee on Nomenclature and Statistics (1980) Diagnostic and Statistical Manual of Mental Disorders. 3rd ed. Washington DC, American Psychiatric Association

Beck AT, Epstein N, Harrison R (1983) Cognitions, attitudes and personality dimensions in depression. Br J Cognitive Psychotherapy 1:1–16

Beck AT, Beck RW (1972) Screening depressed patients in family practice. Postgrad Med 47:81–85

Boyd JH, Burke JD, Gruenberg E, Holzer CE, Rae DS, George LK, Karno M, Stoltzman R, McEvoy L, Nestadt G (1984) Exclusion criteria of DSM-III. Arch Gen Psychiatry 41:983–989

Butler G, Mathews AM (1983) Cognitive processes in anxiety. Adv Beh Res Ther 5:51–62

Cormier SM (1981) A match-mismatch theory of limbic system function. Physiological Psychology 9:3–36

Chambless DL, Caputo GC, Jasin SE, Gracely EJ, Williams C (1985) The mobility inventory for agoraphobia. Beh Res Ther 23:35–44

Gray J (1982) Neuropsychology of anxiety. Oxford University Press, Oxford

Guze RB, Wolfgram ED, McKinney JK, Cantwell DD (1967) Psychiatric illness in the families of convicted criminals: A study of 519 first degree relatives. Dis Nerv Syst 28:651–659

Hibbert GA (1984) Ideational components of anxiety. Br J Psychiatry 144:618–624

Hoehn-Saric R (1981) Characteristics of chronic anxiety patients. In: Klein DF, Rabkin J (eds) Anxiety: New research and changing concepts. Raven Press, New York

Hoehn-Saric R (1982) Comparison of generalized anxiety disorder with panic disorder patients. Psychopharmacol Bull 18:104–108

Katon W (1984) Panic disorder and somatization. Am J Med 77:101–107

Koob GF, Lebrun C, Martinez J, Dantzer R, Le Moal M, Bloom F (1985) Arginine Vasopressin, Stress and Memory. Ann NY Acad Sci 444:194–202

Margraf J, Ehlers A, Roth WT (1986) Sodium lactate infusion and panic attacks: a review and critique. Psychosom Med 48:23–51

Mathews AM, Gelder MG, Johnston DW (1981) Agoraphobia: Nature and treatment. Guilford Press, New York

Mathews AM, MacLeod C (1985) Selective processing of threat cues in anxiety states. Beh Res Ther 23:563–569

Sarter M, Markowitsch HJ (1985) Involvement of the amygdala in learning and memory: A critical review with emphasis on anatomical relations. Behavioral Neuroscience 99:342–380

Stanton ME, Patterson JF, Levine S (1985) Social influences on conditioned cortisol secretion in the squirrel monkey. Psychoneuroendocrinology 10:125–134

Spielberger CD, Gorsuch RL, Lushene RE (1970) STAI Manual. Consulting Psychologist's Press, Palo Alto, California

Spitzer RL, Williams JB (1984) Diagnostic dilemmas. Psychosomatics, Supplement 25:16–20

Thorpe GL, Burns LE (1983) The agoraphobic syndrome. Wiley, Chichester

Tyrer PJ (1973) Relevance of bodily feelings in emotion. Lancet 1973:915–916

Tyrer PJ (1976) The role of bodily feelings in anxiety. Oxford University Press, London

Tyrer PJ, Lee I, Alexander J (1980) Awareness of cardiac function in anxious phobic and hypochondriacal patients. Psychol Med 10:171–174

Section III

Treatments and Longterm Outcome of Phobias with Panic Attacks

9. Longterm Efficacy of Exposure in-Vivo for Cardiac Phobia

Wolfgang Fiegenbaum

1. Introduction

The present study is part of a research program designed to evaluate the efficacy of exposure therapy in phobic disorders. Therapies were conducted between 1977 and 1982 at the universities of Marburg, Münster, and Bonn, West Germany (Bartling et al. 1980a, 1980b; Fiegenbaum 1985). Here we present the treatment outcome of a group of patients suffering from cardiac phobia. According to recent data of Buller et al. (1985), cardiac phobia represents a subgroup of panic disorder as defined by DSM-III (APA 1980). In our research program, 33 cardiac phobics received individual exposure therapy. A subgroup of these patients received additional group sessions of problem solving therapy. This report focuses on the long-term outcome of these treatments at three-year follow-up.

2. Description of our Exposure Therapy Package

The basic approach of exposure therapy is to prevent the patient's avoidance behavior and thus enable him/her to habituate to anxiety-provoking stimuli (Marks 1969, 1972; Birbaumer 1977; Epstein 1977; Bartling et al. 1980b; Fiegenbaum 1982). Further therapeutic components include

I thank Anke Ehlers for help in preparing the manuscript.

the experience of an anxiety decrease in situations that used to be highly anxiety-provoking and the non-occurrence of anticipated threatening events such as cardiac arrest. These processes result in a cognitive reappraisal of the threatening situation.

The therapeutic package designed by our group consisted of four phases (Bartling et al. 1980a).

1. Diagnostic phase
2. Cognitive preparation
3. Intense exposure in vivo
4. Self-control

In the following, we give a description of these different phases.

2.1. Diagnostic Phase

Corresponding to the definition of Richter and Beckmann (1969), we define cardiac phobia as recurrent anxiety attacks in conjunction with the patient's unrealistic fear of suffering from cardiac disease. At the same time, any organic cardiac disorder has to be excluded.

Cardiac phobics closely observe their cardiac function. They tend to avoid situations that lead to physical exertion and might challenge the circulatory system. Furthermore they usually avoid situations in which, in case of an emergency, medical care would not be available. Many of our patients took extreme care to have the addresses of their physicians and coins for the use of public telephones with them.

For all patients in this study we collected information necessary for planning and conducting the flooding therapy. This included:

1. situational and reaction-specific characteristics of the cardiac phobic,
2. type and degree of avoidance behavior,
3. the patient's motivation,
4. evaluation of the problem by significant others,
5. facilitating and inhibiting conditions in the patient's social environment and economic situation.

2.2. Cognitive Preparation

We consider cognitive preparation, which takes place a few days prior to the intense exposure sessions, a central component of our treatment package. The goal is to explain the development and maintenance of phobic avoidance behavior and to make the course of therapy transparent and understandable for the patient. Furthermore, therapeutic rapport is established and the patient is prepared for making an independent decision to participate in the program.

First of all, the therapist presents an easily comprehendable model of the etiology of cardiac phobia to the patient which is based on Mowrer's two-factor theory (Mowrer 1960). Examples from the patient's own history are used to show the role of hypochondriacal self-observation of cardiac sensations and, most important, the role of avoidance in the maintenance of anxiety. Subsequently, the therapist explains how treatment will resolve cardiac phobia by prolonged exposure and habituation to various anxiety-provoking situations.

We consider the patient's (self-determined) commitment to participate in the therapy of central importance for therapeutic outcome. To enable patients to make such an independent decision, they are given several days without any further intervention from the therapist after completion of the cognitive preparation phase.

2.3. Intense Exposure in-Vivo

The basic idea of in vivo training is for patients to expose themselves to anxiety-provoking situations as long as is necessary to experience the situation without any anxiety. Training lasts several days and tackles as many different situations as possible. For this purpose, daily training sessions of six to eight hours duration are held in the patient's natural environment. To elicit anxiety, the patient is exposed to highly anxiety-provoking situations that were carefully planned and specified prior to the session. The therapist strictly prevents behavioral and cognitive attempts to escape or avoid the situation. The patient is instructed to concentrate on the 'here and now' of the situation and on his/her cardiac sensations. The time the patient needs to reach a substantial decrease in anxiety, determines the duration of exposure to the individual situation. Apart from a few exceptions, this usually takes no more than 20–30 min. It is essential that the patient stays in the situation without any cognitive distraction and without any relief from medication.

By exposing the patient sequentially to various highly anxiety-provoking situations, he/she will experience rapid success. Also, habituation is facilitated by physical exhaustion (Birbaumer 1977).

The therapist closely supervises the first few sequences of training. Then, a step-wise transition to a self-controlled training program is introduced.

2.4. Self-Control

The self-control phase is introduced when the therapist is certain that the patient does not show any further escape or avoidance behavior. Patient and therapist discuss the next situation to be tackled by the patient. An agreement is made that the patient uses the same principles as in the intense exposure phase (that is, to concentrate on the situation and the cardiac sensations without any distraction, and to stay in the situation until he/she is free of anxiety). Special emphasis is given to the role of cognitive avoidance strategies.

At the end of the self-control phase, therapist and patient discuss the experiences made in this phase. Furthermore, a framework for subsequent training (situations, time fram and frequency) for stabilization of therapeutic gains is agreed upon.

3. Goals and Design of our Study

Our study assessed the long-term effects of the exposure therapy package described above in a group of patients with cardiac phobia. Another goal was to determine whether additional group therapy would enhance therapeutic outcome and lead to better stability of treatment effects. The group therapy used a problem-solving approach. Groups addressed problems that had a probable functional connection to the cardiac phobia (Grawe 1980; Chambless 1982; Fiegenbaum 1985).

Twenty patients received the treatment package described above (group A). The average duration of treatment (contact with the therapist) was 20 hours. Thirteen patients received an additional 20 hours of problem-solving group therapy following the exposure therapy (group B). Figure 1 shows the study design.

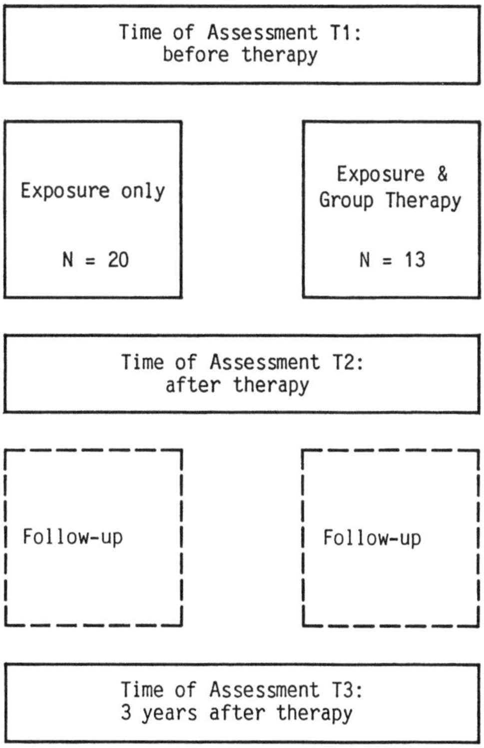

Fig. 1. Study design

4. Methods

4.1. Patients and Therapists

A total of thirty-three patients with a diagnosis of cardiac phobia were referred by physicians in private practice (general and internal medicine), university hospitals, and counseling centers. According to DSM-III, our patients would have been diagnosed as suffering from agoraphobia with panic attacks.

Table 1 shows the demographic characteristics of our patient sample. The majority of patients were females. We chose to study a relatively homogeneous group of patients. Furthermore, the group therapy sessions focused on problems typically experienced by female patients. Patients had a mean age of 34 years, 60.6% were married, and only 21.3% were gainfully employed. The average duration of symptoms was 7.7 years. 84.8% had received prior treatment for their cardiac phobia.

Individual and group sessions were conducted by two co-therapists. Therapists were graduate students in clinical psychology who had passed the clinical curriculum and had received additional training in the treatment package described above (cf. Fiegenbaum 1985).

4.2. Assessment

In this report we focus on symptom-oriented measures that assessed the quality and degree of the patient's behavioral and cognitive-emotional responses to the phobic situation. The assessment schedule is found in Fig. 1. Assessment 1 (T1) took place before treatment, assessment 2 (T2) after the end of treatment, and assessment 3 (T3) three years after the end of treatment.

Table 1. Overview of the demographic data

	Entire group		Group A		Group B	
Number of subjects (N)	33		20		13	
Age (mean)	34.5		33.7		35.2	
Duration of symptoms ($\bar{x}$) in months	91.9		91.0		93.4	
	%	N	%	N	%	N
Gender						
Male	6.1	2	10.0	2	–	–
Female	93.9	31	90.0	18	100	13
Family status						
Single	30.3	10	30.0	6	30.8	4
Married	60.6	20	60.0	12	61.5	8
Widowed	9.1	3	10.0	2	7.7	1
Education						
9 years	54.5	18	10.0	2	23.1	3
11 years	21.2	7	25.0	5	15.4	2
13 years	15.2	5	10.0	2	23.1	3
University degree	9.1	3	10.0	2	7.7	1
Previous treatment						
Yes	84.8	28	85.0	17	84.6	11
No	15.2	5	15.0	3	15.4	2

Group A = exposure therapy only
Group B = combined exposure and group therapy

4.2.1. Questionnaire Measures

(a) Global rating (Glob) on an anxiety thermometer
The patient is asked to rate the degree of his/her cardiac anxiety on a scale from 0 (totally anxiety-free) to 100 (maximum anxiety imaginable). We asked the patient to rate the three situations on this scale that he/she described as the most anxiety-provoking in the initial interview. The global anxiety rating (Glob) is the sum of the scores for these three situations.

(b) Situation Rating Scale (SB)
The SB-scale (Ullrich and Ullrich de Muynck 1979) was especially developed to assess the efficacy of anxiety treatments. Its validity has been established. The scale assesses several dimensions of the cognitive appraisal of anxiety-provoking situations, of behavioral tendencies, of expectancies about the consequences of one's own behavior as well as a self-description of the patient. The questionnaire is a polarity profile of 55 pairs of adjectives. The patient is asked to describe his/her phobic situation on six-point Lickert scales. Factor analyses resulted in six factors such as avoidance tendency and degree of perceived threat.

(c) Emotionality Inventory (EMI-S)
The EMI-S (Ullrich and Ullrich de Muynck 1979) assesses the patient's emotional state in response to the phobic situation. The questionnaire consists of 70 pairs of adjectives. The patient is asked to describe his subjective state on six-point Lickert scales. The authors found seven interpretable factors of sufficient eigenvalue such as anxious-inhibited vs. relaxed-secure reaction or exhausted-passive vs. dynamic-active reaction.

The variables EMI-S1 (anxious) and EMI-S5 (optimistic) could not be included in the analyses since a preliminary version of the scale was used in the first patient groups that had another factor structure (cf. Fiegenbaum 1985).

4.2.2. Behavioral Test

At the 3 year follow-up, a behavioral test was conducted. The patient was asked to expose him/herself to the situation which had been rated as most anxiety-provoking at the beginning of therapy. This test was explicitly not a repetition of a therapeutic session; patients could leave the situation at any time or could refuse to enter the situation at all. The behavioral test was recorded on video tape. Independent observers trained in the use of a structured observation schedule rated the tapes for cardiac phobic symptoms on the behavioral and cognitive-emotional levels.

4.2.3. Other Symptom-Relevant Variables

In addition, we assessed the following variables relevant to the patient's cardiac phobia by questionnaires or structured interviews.

(a) Protocols of medication use, evaluated by a pharmacologist,
(b) degree of disability in private and professional environment,
(c) occupation,
(d) occurrence of panic attacks,
(e) other medical treatment and psychotherapy.

5. Results

We will first present the results for the entire patient group (N = 33), that is group A (exposure therapy only, N = 20) and group B (exposure therapy plus problem solving group therapy, N = 13). Secondly, we will present a comparison of the two groups.

5.1. Results for the Entire Patient Group

5.1.1. Questionnaire Measures

Multivariate Hotelling T^2 tests were used to test therapeutic outcome in twelve variables obtained from the three questionnaires described above (Glob, EMI-S, SB). When appropriate, post-hoc t-tests were used to test in which of the variables chang-

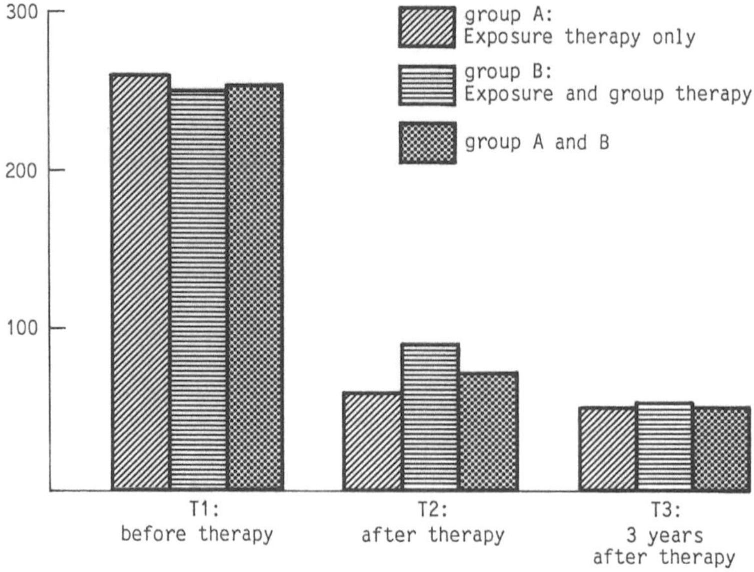

Fig. 2. Global rating of intensity of cardiac anxiety at assessments T1, T2, and T3. Means of the subject groups A and B as well as of the entire group are presented

Table 2. Entire patient group; symptom-oriented measures at assessments T1, T2, T3

Group (N)	A+B (33)	A+B (33)	A+B (33)
Time of assessment	T1/T2	T2/T3	T1/T3
Multivariate (F)	952.28***	1.58	882.15***
Univariate (t)			
GLOB	8.84***	2.09	19.45***
SB 1	7.32***	5.32**	6.53***
SB 2	6.31***	0.08	12.08***
SB 3	9.25***	1.14	8.14***
SB 4	−5.41***	−2.21	−1.56
SB 5	0.71	1.16	4.15*
SB 6	−3.03*	−0.91	−4.15*
EMI-S 2	5.89***	2.24	9.84***
EMI-S 3	11.41***	1.89	7.52***
EMI-S 4	6.58***	1.88	6.84***
EMI-S 6	−7.54***	−1.76	9.31***
EMI-S 7	12.58***	1.45	7.59***
In favor of	T2		T3

* $p < 0.05$; ** $p < 0.01$; *** $p < 0.001$
A = Exposure therapy only
B = Combined exposure and group therapy
T1 = Before therapy
T2 = After therapy
T3 = Three years after end of therapy

es had occurred. Table 2 shows the results for these measures.

The multivariate comparison of T1 and T3, that is assessment before therapy compared with the assessment three years after the end of therapy, showed a significant improvement in the symptom-oriented questionnaire measures ($p < 0.001$). Univariate post-hoc tests (t-tests) showed improvements for almost all of the variables. The same applies to the comparison of T1 and T2, that is assessment before therapy compared to the end of therapy ($p < 0.001$ for the multivariate comparison). During follow-up (T2 compared with T3), no significant changes were observed. Improvement remained stable. Fig. 2 illustrates the time course of changes for the variable Glob, which is typical for the other 11 variables as well.

5.1.2. Behavioral Test

At the three year follow-up, 27 of 33 patients (81.8%) mastered the situation that used to be most anxiety-provoking before therapy without any problems. Four patients (12.1%) refused to enter the situation, two (6.1%) left the situation early. Those

Table 3. Groups A and B; other symptom-relevant variables before and 3 years after therapy

Group (N)	A and B (33)				A (20)				B (13)			
	Before therapy		3 year follow-up		Before therapy		3 year follow-up		Before therapy		3 year follow-up	
	%	N	%	N	%	N	%	N	%	N	%	N
Occupation												
Full-time	12.1	4	33.3	11	10.0	2	30.0	6	15.4	2	38.5	5
Part-time	18.2	6	24.2	8	10.0	2	20.0	4	30.8	4	30.8	4
None	69.7	23	42.4	14	80.0	16	50.0	10	53.8	7	30.8	4
Use of medications												
Yes	75.8	25	15.2	5	80.0	16	10.0	2	69.2	9	23.1	3
No	24.2	8	84.8	28	20.0	4	90.0	18	30.8	4	76.9	10
Fear of leaving house												
Yes	63.6	21	6.1	2	75.0	15	10.0	2	46.2	6	0.0	0
No	36.4	12	93.9	31	25.0	5	90.0	18	53.8	7	100.0	13

Group A = Exposure therapy only
Group B = Combined exposure and group therapy

patients who mastered the situation showed very little avoidance behavior. Motor behavior and observable physiological responses indicated little anxiety. The patients reported that they mastered the situation nearly anxiety-free.

5.1.3. Other Symptom-Relevant Variables

In a structured interview, patients reported that they had no or very few panic attacks during follow-up. Only five (15.2%) had sought additional treatment due to difficulties with the partner (three patients), depression, hypertension and obesity (one patient each). No patient had sought additional treatment for her/his cardiac phobia.

Table 3 shows the results for three other variables. At the three year follow-up, two patients (6.1%) were unable to leave their homes compared to 21 (63.6%) prior to treatment. In addition, there was a non-significant trend for an increase in employment rate. Furthermore, medication use was decreased.

Table 4. Group A; symptom-oriented measures at assessments T1, T2, T3

Group (N)	A (20)	A (20)	A (20)
Time of assessment	T1/T2	T2/T3	T1/T3
Multivariate (F)	908.61**	9.85	889.92***
Univariate (t)			
GLOB	8.89***	0.71	6.95***
SB 1	11.86***	0.95	8.64***
SB 2	5.45***	1.61	6.51***
SB 3	7.52***	3.67**	9.51***
SB 4	−3.67**	−1.11	−3.65**
SB 5	1.51	1.48	1.71
SB 6	−3.31*	0.09	−2.78*
EMI-S 2	8.52***	1.71	9.57***
EMI-S 3	4.61***	0.65	5.89***
EMI-S 4	6.51***	0.21	8.03***
EMI-S 6	−8.90***	−0.41	−7.53***
EMI-S 7	5.91***	−0.11	6.14***
In favor of	T2		T3

* $p < 0.05$; ** $p < 0.01$; *** $p < 0.001$
A = Exposure therapy only
T1 = Before therapy
T2 = After therapy
T3 = Three years after end of therapy

Table 5. Group B; symptom-oriented measures at assessments T1, T2, T3

Group (N)	B (13)	B (13)	B (13)
Time of assessment	T1/T2	T2/T3	T1/T3
Multivariate (F)	27.41*	1.98	221.30*
Univariate (t)			
GLOB	8.82***	1.89	19.49***
SB 1	4.90***	1.85	9.51***
SB 2	3.38**	2.68*	11.30***
SB 3	5.15***	3.58**	7.95***
SB 4	−3.41**	−1.08	−3.45**
SB 5	0.48	1.15	1.16
SB 6	−2.48*	0.18	−2.41*
EMI-S 2	5.22***	0.04	7.41***
EMI-S 3	3.61**	1.01	9.98***
EMI-S 4	5.28***	0.09	2.95*
EMI-S 6	−4.35**	1.21	−11.17***
EMI-S 7	2.46*	0.78	5.15**
In favor of	T2		T3

* $p < 0.05$; ** $p < 0.01$; *** $p < 0.001$
B = Combined exposure and group therapy
T1 = Before therapy
T2 = After therapy
T3 = Three years after end of therapy

5.2. Comparison of Groups A and B

Tables 4 and 5 show the results for the questionnaire measures for group A (exposure therapy only) and group B (combination of exposure therapy and group therapy), respectively. The results were very similar and are parallel to those described for the entire patient group.

Table 6 shows the comparison of groups A and B. The groups did not differ in their baseline scores. Comparison of T1 and T2 (therapy phase) showed a larger improvement for group A ($p < 0.05$ for the multivariate analysis). Thus, at the end of therapy, group A that had only received flooding therapy was less symptomatic than group B that had received the combination of treatments ($p < 0.05$ for the multivariate comparison). However, group B showed larger gains during the follow-up phase (T2 vs. T3, $p < 0.05$ for the multivariate comparison). At the 3 year follow-up, no significant differences between the groups were observed.

Table 6. Group A versus B; symptom-oriented measures at assessments T1, T2, T3

Group (N)	A vs B (20/13)					
Time of assessment	T1	T1/T2	T2	T2/T3	T3	T1/T3
Multivariate (F)	1.15	2.26	2.53	2.31	0.98	1.28
Univariate (t) GLOB	1.33	2.98	21.16***	4.64*	0.61	2.21
SB 1	−1.72	4.01*	11.54***	3.75*	0.38	1.68
SB 2	−0.90	11.38***	13.31***	2.08	1.24	1.33
SB 3	−0.98	7.18**	16.95***	3.49*	0.16	2.08
SB 4	1.34	1.16	19.31***	2.87	0.99	0.69
SB 5	0.08	0.31	5.98**	5.32**	1.11	0.91
SB 6	0.50	3.31*	17.11***	4.68*	0.68	3.72*
EMI-S 2	−1.16	3.98*	12.96***	3.62*	3.40*	2.04
EMI-S 3	0.21	4.08*	7.03**	2.28	2.80	0.31
EMI-S 4	−0.04	3.32*	2.08	1.89	0.01	0.83
EMI-S 6	0.31	6.98**	9.51***	3.81*	0.23	0.95
EMI-S 7	1.11	7.03***	11.58***	5.36**	0.94	1.08
In favor of		A	A	B	–	–

* $p < 0.05$; ** $p < 0.01$; *** $p < 0.001$
A = Exposure therapy
B = Combined exposure and group therapy
T1 = Before therapy
T2 = After therapy
T3 = Three years after end of therapy

6. Discussion

The main goal of this study was to assess the long-term efficacy of exposure therapy in patients with cardiac phobic complaints. The results for 33 patients (entire patient group) show a clear improvement during therapy. Gains remained stable during the three year follow-up phase. Improvement was found on questionnaire measures of cardiac phobic complaints and phobic avoidance as well as on a behavioral test. Nearly all of the patients treated in our program no longer show avoidance behavior. They are able to enter situations that used to elicit high anxiety. In the same situation, they are now free of anxiety and somatic complaints. Moreover, patients reported that they did not suffer from panic attacks any more. At the same time, medication use was dramatically decreased.

Problem-solving therapy did not lead to any additional gains. We interpret this result as demonstrating the high efficacy of exposure therapy in the treatment of avoidance behavior. We consider this the essential goal in the treatment of agoraphobia and cardiac phobia. Additional group therapy that is designed to help the patient solve problems related to his/her symptoms does not add much to symptomatic improvement.

If the time course of changes is taken into account (Table 6), the combined treatment group showed a delay in therapeutic gains. We hypothesize that the problem solving group therapy taught the patients a more complex view of their problems, which might have led them to evaluate the therapeutic effect of therapy more critically. The results from other assessment points not discussed here, however, showed that the relative advantage of exposure therapy ended shortly after the end of therapy (T2). Both treatment groups showed the same stability of treatment outcome during the follow-up phase (T2 to T3).

7. References

American Psychiatric Association, committee on Nomenclature and Statistics (1980) Diagnostic and Statistical Manual of Mental Disorders. 3rd ed. Washington DC, American Psychiatric Association

Bartling G (1982) Bericht über eine problemorientierte Gruppentherapie. In: Fiegenbaum W (ed) Psychologische Therapie in der Praxis. Kohlhammer, Stuttgart

Bartling G, Fiegenbaum W, Krause R (1980a) Reizüberflutung. Theorie und Praxis. Kohlhammer, Stuttgart

Bartling G, Fiegenbaum W, Krause R (1980b) Einige Überlegungen zu kognitiven Grundlagen der Reizüberflutung. Zeitschr f Klin Psychol 9:235–244

Birbaumer N (1977) (ed) Psychophysiologie der Angst. Urban & Schwarzenberg, München (Fortschritte der klinischen Psychologie Bd 3)

Buller R, Maier W, Knisel M (1985) Herzangstsyndrom – ein Subtyp der Panikattacken. Paper presented at the 15th Annual Meeting of the EABT, Munich

Butollo W (1979) Chronische Angst: Theorie und Praxis der Konfrontationstherapie. Urban & Schwarzenberg, München

Chambless DL (1982) Characteristics of agoraphobics. In: Chambless DL, Goldstein AJ (eds) Agoraphobia. Multiple perspectives on theory and treatment. Wiley, New York

Epstein S (1977) Versuch einer Theorie der Angst. In: Birbaumer N (ed) Psychophysiologie der Angst. Urban & Schwarzenberg, München, pp 208–266

Fiegenbaum W (1982) Konfrontationsverfahren. In: Bastine R (ed) Grundbegriffe der Psychotherapie. Beltz, Weinheim

Fiegenbaum W (1985) Agoraphobie – Theoretische Konzepte und Behandlungsmethoden. Westdeutscher Verlag, Wiesbaden

Grawe K (1980) (ed) Verhaltenstherapie in Gruppen. Urban & Schwarzenberg, München

Marks IM (1969) Fears and phobias. Heinemann, London

Marks IM (1972) Flooding and allied treatments. In: Agras WS (ed) Behavior modification, principles and clinical applications. Little Brown Co., Boston

Mowrer OH (1960) Learning theory and behavior. Wiley, New York

Richter HE, Beckmann D (1969) Herzneurose. Thieme, Stuttgart

Ullrich R, Ullrich de Muynck R (1979) Das Situationsbewertungssystem SB-EMI-S. Anleitung für den Therapeuten Teil III. Pfeiffer, München

10. Cognitive and Physiological Processes in the Maintainance and Treatment of Panic Attacks

Paul M. Salkovskis and David M. Clark

1. Introduction

Panic attacks are defined as sudden onset episodes of intense anxiety accompanied by a range of unpleasant bodily sensations (American Psychiatric Association 1980). Patients report that cognitions accompanying such attacks commonly concern ideas of going mad, having a heart attack or other acute medical emergency, or of losing control of their behaviour in such a way as to disgrace themselves (Beck, Laude and Bohnert 1974; Hibbert 1984). Panic attacks occur in both phobic and non-phobic anxiety states. In the former case, it has been argued that the fear of such panic attacks may be responsible for the avoidance behaviour which plays such a prominent part in agoraphobia (Goldstein and Chambless 1978).

Authorship is equal. The authors are grateful to the Medical Research Council of the United Kingdom for its support.

Acknowledgements: The authors would like to thank Jack Chalkley, David Jones, Hilary Warwick and Julie Wessels who contributed to the studies described here; also, Pergamon Press for permission to reproduce Figures 2, 3 and 8; the Royal College of Psychiatrists for permission to reproduce Figures 4 and 5, and John Libby (publishers) for permission to reproduce Figures 6 and 7.

Many writers have commented on the similarity between the physical symptoms of panic attacks and those produced by hyperventilation (Clark 1979; Clark and Hemsley 1982; Kerr, Dalton and Gliebe 1937; Lum 1976). This similarity, together with the observation that hyperventilation may occur as a consequence of anxiety (Seuss, Alexander, Smith, Sweeney and Marion 1980) has led to the suggestion that hyperventilation may play an important part in the production of panic attacks. It should, however, be noted that there are considerable individual differences in the affective response to hyperventilation (Clark and Hemsley 1982; Svebak and Grossman 1985), such that some individuals may experience the sensations produced by overbreathing as pleasurable, whilst others find them unpleasant or frightening. Such differences in response appear to be mediated by factors such as personality and the context in which similar sensations have previously been experienced. Thus, hyperventilation *per se* does not cause panic attacks. Instead, it has been hypothesised (Clark 1986) that hyperventilation only leads to panic if the sensations which it produces are interpreted in a catastrophic fashion. The specific way in which hyperventilation may contribute to the production of panic attacks in individuals prone to catastrophically interpret bodily sensations is illustrated in Fig. 1.

A wide range of stimuli may trigger attacks; such stimuli may be external (for example, situations in which previous attacks have been experienced) or internal (bodily sensations, frightening thoughts or images). If these stimuli are perceived as threatening, apprehension results. In many individuals, such apprehension is accompanied by increased ventilation which in turn produces a drop in $paCO_2$ and increased pH. This leads to a wide range of bodily and CNS symptoms such as dizziness, shakiness, numbness of extremities, tachycardia, palpitations, nausea, breathlessness and feelings of faintness. Further apprehension results from the experience (or intensification) of these sensations if they are themselves interpreted in a catastrophic fashion. They may also augment the fear already elicited by other stimuli by a process of inappropriate labelling, as in the Schachter and Singer (1962) experiments. Apprehension would be expected to lead to a further increase in ventilation, and so on round in a vicious circle. Furthermore, the most severe anxiety would be expected amongst those in whom the catastrophes they fear are thought to be imminent (i.e. likely to occur in the next few moments) or to have already started. It is not difficult to appreciate the difference between the individual who responds to feelings of breathlessness, faintness and palpitations by the thought "I'm having a heart attack just like my father did" as opposed to "I've been overdoing things lately, and I'm exhausted." Cognitions consequent on otherwise similar bodily sensations may thus vary considerably between individuals and are likely to have considerable impact on the amount of anxiety experienced.

Appraisal of helplessness in the face of panic attacks is likely to lead to further problems and the development of functionally autonomous "fear of the consequences of fear"; i.e. the belief that anxiety itself may serve to trigger the disastrous consequences anticipated and that there is little they can do during an attack to avert this. The development of apparently maladaptive avoidance behaviours intended to

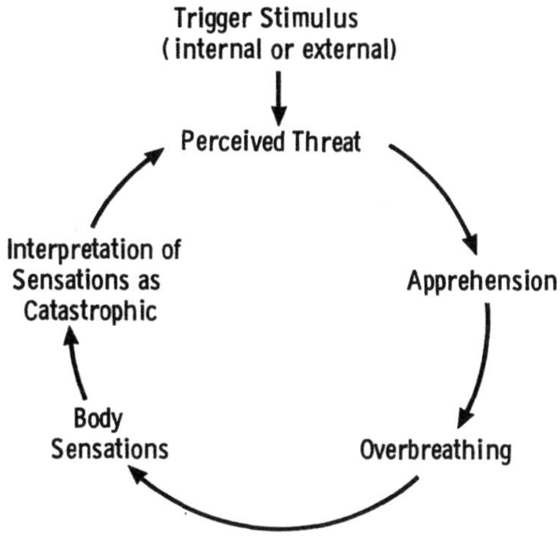

Fig. 1. A schematic representation of the short-term interaction between cognitive and physiological mechanisms in hyperventilation-related panic attacks

avoid the possibility of having attacks (and therefore avert the feared catastrophes) would be expected to increase this sensitivity yet more. Repeated and prolonged overbreathing results in renal excretion of bicarbonate and hence a reset of the blood buffer systems (Gibson 1978). Such changes produce enhanced responsiveness to even quite small changes in $paCO_2$ and hence a lowered threshold for the development of symptoms of overbreathing, so that very mild stressors (such as excitement or exercise) may lead to symptoms. Thus, both short and longer term changes in cognitions, behaviour and physiology are involved, and are liable to interact in quite complicated ways.

It should be noted that the above model of the role of hyperventilation in panic attacks is a specific example of a more general cognitive model of panic (Clark 1986). As discussed in Clark (1986), this model is able to account for the major features of panic, including the occurrence of "spontaneous" panic attacks. It is argued that such attacks are, triggered by bodily sensations or frightening thoughts which immediately precede an attack but are perceived as part of it. Patients' response to pharmacological "panic inductions" (such as infusions of lactate or inhalations of CO_2) can also be accounted for by the model. Here it is hypothesised that patients' affective response to the procedures is mediated by the interpretations which patients make of the bodily sensations which are produced by the inductions. Both the occurrence of spontaneous attacks and the effectiveness of pharmacological induction procedures have previously been taken as strong support for a biological model, in which panic is regarded as a form of "endogeneous anxiety". The present paper describes a series of investigations into panic attacks, which were derived from the model shown in Fig. 1.

The first set of studies investigated the effects of a cognitive behavioural treatment of panic which was derived from the model. In particular, it was hypothesised that panic could be treated effectively by:

1. The appropriate reattribution of the sensations experienced during panic attacks to hyperventilation and away from catastrophic interpretations.
2. Modifying respiratory and cognitive responses to stress.

The second set of investigations addressed the question of whether patients who experienced panic attacks in which symptoms characteristic of hyperventilation are prominent actually increase ventilation (a) under stress resembling that which precipitates their panic attacks (b) during naturally occurring panic attacks.

2. Effectiveness of Treatment Based on the Cognitive Model of Panic

Patients treated in both of the studies described were routine referrals to Departments of Clinical Psychology; all experienced frequent panic attacks. "Situationals" who reported that there were certain situations in which they consistently experienced anxiety were analysed seperately from "non-situationals", who were unable to identify such consistency in their anxiety. In the first study, patients were selected on the basis that there was some evidence on assessment to suggest that hyperventilation may play a role in their panic attacks, whereas patients in the second study were unselected to allow investigation of the role of such a similarity in predicting outcome. In both studies the experimental design was similar, with a no treatment baseline followed by an intensive intervention directed at illustrating to the patient the link between respiration, cognitions and the symptoms which they experienced during panic attacks. In both investigations, the design strategy employed was to establish a stable baseline and assess the impact of the intervention in a shorter period than the baseline. A significant effect within this period can confidently be attributed to the intervention itself rather than to spontaneous remission, but the design does not allow any appraisal of the effective elements of treatment. Several treatment procedures were used (a brief period of forced ventilation designed to reproduce the bodily sensations experienced during panic if they were hyperventilation related; reviewing the patients perception of this test in the context of the sequence of events in naturally occurring panic) to provide an initial basis for the reattribution of the symptoms the patients experienced to stress induced hyperventilation. Patients invariably viewed such an explanation as much less catastrophic than the things which they had previously feared (e.g. heart attacks, going mad, having a stroke, epileptic fits). Practice in respiratory control and more appropriate cognitive responses to anxiety symptoms were then provided and patients were encouraged to use these strategies to control panic and so provide further evidence for the validity of non-catastrophic interpretations of their symptoms. Following a period of this intervention (during which time the patients were asked not to go into situations which they had previously avoided), graded exposure was commenced for those patients who showed marked phobic avoidance.

In both studies, measures included a daily diary of panic attack frequency, behavioural avoidance tests where appropriate, Marks and Mathews (1979) Fear Questionnaire and the Beck Depression Inventory (Beck and Beamsderfer 1974). In the second study, extra measures were added: daily diary of panic severity and ratings of generalised anxiety, and a modification of the rebreathing method of measurement of pCO_2 (Cambell and Howell 1962).

Study 1 (Clark, Salkovskis and Chalkley 1985):

Panic attacks: Figure 2 shows the mean number of panic attacks per week for situationals and non situationals. A repeated measures ANOVA (situational/non-situational as grouping factor, time of testing as repeated measures within subjects) showed a significant effect of time, $p < 0.01$. Newman Keuls tests indicated that patients experienced significantly less panic attacks by week 2 of "pure" respiratory treatment than in any week of the baseline. (Significance levels of all ANOVA's were tested using the Greenhouse Geisser correction (epsilon) for serially dependent data (Keselman and Rogan 1980)). A significant linear trend for time indicated that improvement continued between weeks 2 and 13.

Behaviour Test: Figure 3 shows the patients self-rated anxiety during two pretreatment and a post-treatment behaviour test.

There was no significant difference between the two pretreatment tests, indicating that the test itself did not have a therapeutic effect. The patients rated themselves as significantly less anxious during the post-treatment test, indicating that a few days of pure respiratory control treatment had had the effect of reducing situational anxiety.

Fear Questionnaire: Results on this indicated that, as predicted, patients did not show a significant reduction in avoidance during the "pure" respiratory phase, but that there was a significant reduction in

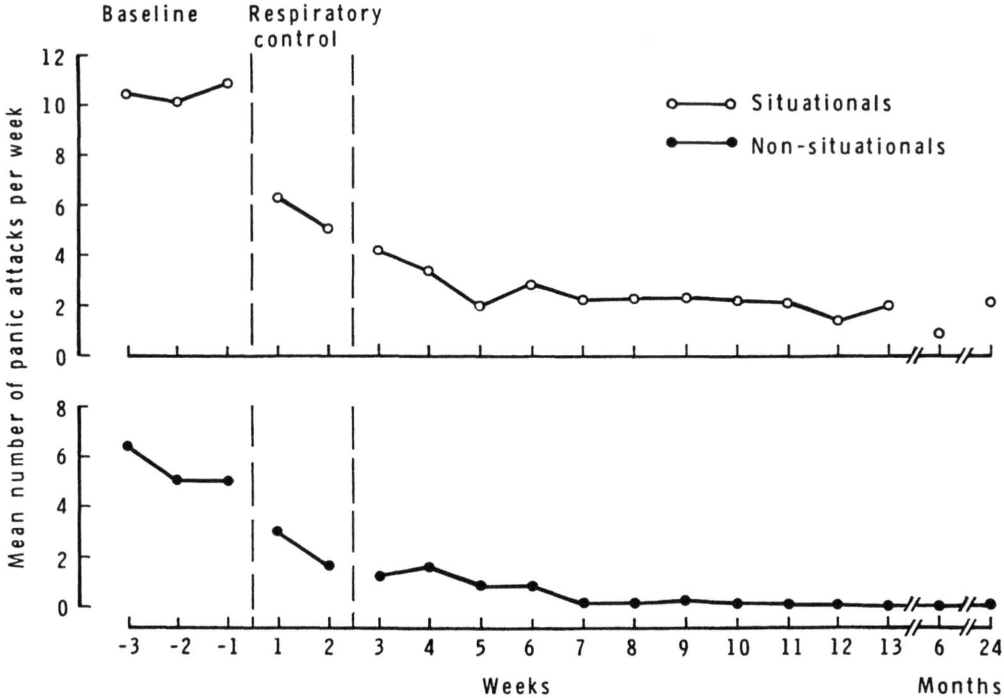

Fig. 2. Frequency of panic attacks per week for situational and non-situational groups in study 1 (self rating from daily diary). (Reproduced with permission from Clark, Salkovskis and Chalkley (1985) Respiratory control as a treatment for panic attacks. J. Behav. Ther. and Exp. Psychiat. **13,** Pergamon Press.)

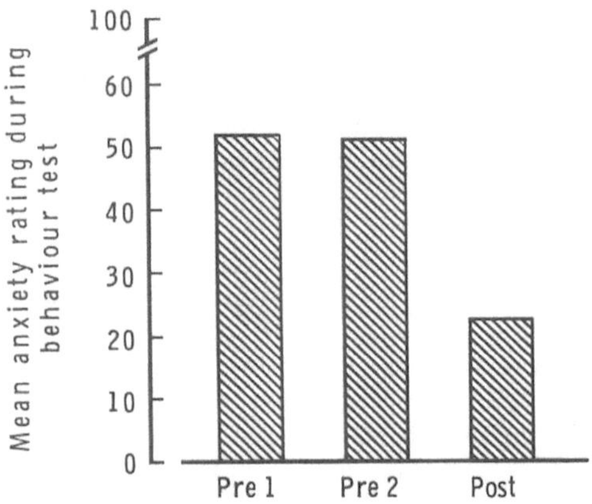

Fig. 3. Self ratings of anxiety during the behaviour test. (Reproduced with permission from Clark, Salkovskis and Chalkley (1985) Respiratory control as a treatment for panic attacks. J. Behav. Ther. and Exp. Psychiat. **13,** Pergamon Press.)

avoidance thereafter, making it likely that therapeutic reduction in panic frequency had been brought about by the initial intervention and was not secondary to a reduced level of avoidance. Anxiety/depression and global rating of distress showed immediate and significant reductions with respiratory training, again as predicted.

Beck Depression Inventory: There were no significant effects of treatments on Depression Scores.

Results of this study indicate that the intervention had an immediate effect on panic attack frequency and situational anxiety (Self ratings during behaviour test) which are unlikely to be attributable to changes in exposure, and were maintained for 2 years.

Study 2 (Salkovskis, Jones and Clark 1986): The results of the second study replicated those of the first in all important respects. Figure 4a shows the effect on panic frequency of respiratory control treatment compared with 4 weeks baseline. By the second week of respiratory control, patients were experiencing significantly less panic attacks than during any week of the baseline period.

The daily rating of general anxiety was also analysed in this study; Fig. 4b illustrates the results of this analysis. ANOVA revealed a significant effect of time ($p < 0.05$), and Newman-Keuls tests indicated that patients ratings of generalised anxiety at the fourth week of respiratory control treatment were significantly lower than all four weeks of baseline.

Inspection of ratings of panic attack severity indicated that treatment was associated with a decrease in severity of panic attacks, as well as with reduced frequency. Mean panic attack severity was 51 during the baseline period, dropping to 42 during the first week of respiratory control ($t_d = 4.62$, $p < 0.01$). As respiratory control reduces the severity of panic attacks, it could be argued that Fig. 4a (frequency of attacks) underestimates the effectiveness of the treatment. A fairer estimate may be Fig. 4c, which plots the effects of treatment on Frequency × Severity.

Questionnaire data showed the same results as in the previous study, with the important exception that the avoidance ratings on the Fear Questionnaire showed a significant decrease at the end of four weeks of "pure" respiratory control treatment. In order to assess whether this change could account for the decrease in panic attacks observed, a covariance analysis with change in avoidance scores as covariate was performed for the panic attack data. Significance levels were not changed by this procedure, supporting the view that the observed changes in panic could not be attributed to an increase in exposure.

Measures of pCO_2: The major difference between the second study and the first was the addition of measurement of pCO_2. The stability of the pCO_2 measure used (a modified Cambell and Howell rebreathing technique; full details in Clark 1979) was assessed. Intercorrelations within and between sessions were 0.87 or better; there were no changes in mean resting values observed with repeated measurements. Figure 5 shows resting pCO_2 levels for all patients throughout treatment, together with a reference line indicating mean resting pCO_2 in a group of 23 normal subjects, matched for age and sex. Prior to treatment there is a highly significant ($t_i = 5.57$, $p < 0.01$) difference between patients and controls.

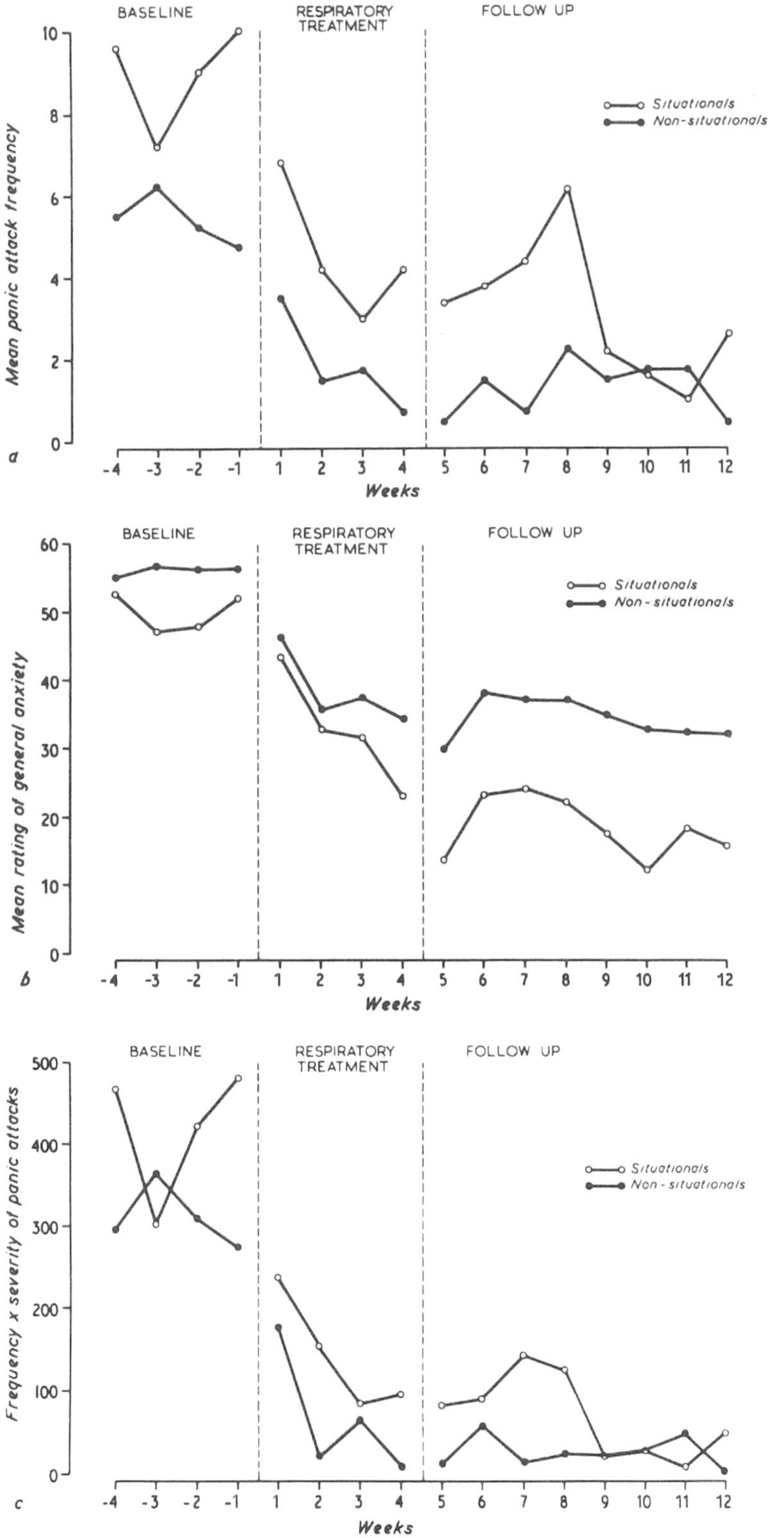

Fig. 4. Self ratings of panic frequency, general anxiety and panic severity × frequency for situational and non-situational groups in study 2 (self rating from daily diary). (From Salkovskis, Jones and Clark 1986; reproduced with permission.)

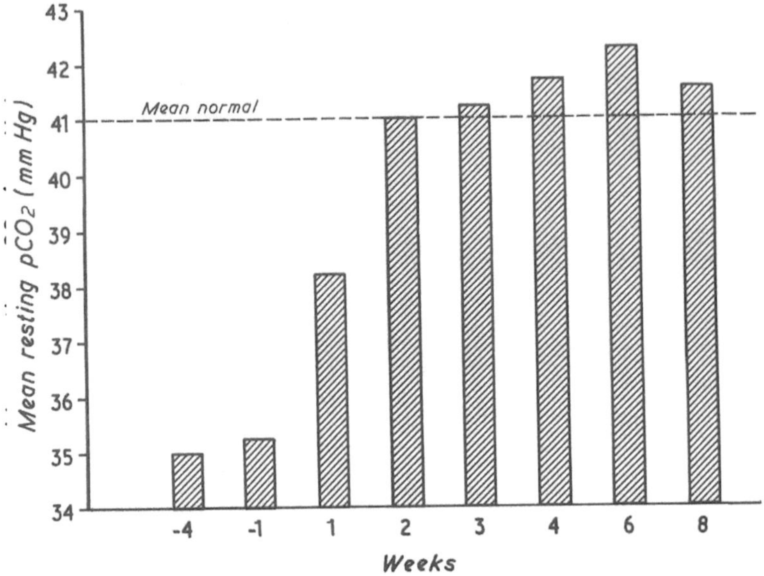

Fig. 5. Resting pCO_2 in study 2 patients throughout treatment (vertical bars) and mean resting pCO_2 in a group of age- and sex-matched controls (horizontal reference line). All values corrected to give $paCO_2$. (From Salkovskis, Jones and Clark 1986; reproduced with permission.)

Within patients resting pCO_2 is significantly higher by the end of the first week of respiratory treatment than during baseline. By the second week of treatment, patients and normals have similar resting levels of pCO_2. Correlational analysis indicated that patients with initially low resting pCO_2 were highly likely to recognise the symptoms of overbreathing as similar to their panic attacks (pCO_2 with similarity: $r=-0.81$, $p<0.01$). Also, recognition of such similarity correlated highly with treatment outcome as measured by changes in Marks and Mathews questionnaire Global rating ($r=0.81$, $p<0.01$); Anxiety/depression ratings ($r=0.66$, $p<0.05$) and total avoidance score ($r=0.76$, $p<0.01$).

3. Interpretation of Treatment Studies

It is unlikely that the observed improvements were due to spontaneous remission as, in both studies, a stable baseline was established, and significant improvements took place in a shorter period than the baseline itself. It is therefore possible to argue that the cognitive-behavioural treatment employed was an effective treatment for panic; this is particularly so when patients perceive a marked similarity between the effects of a period of brief forced ventilation and their naturally occurring panic attacks. Furthermore, patients who perceived such a similarity were more likely to have a lowered resting level of pCO_2. Both observations provide indirect support for the view that hyperventilation might play an important role in the panic attacks experienced by some patients. However, they cannot be taken as strong evidence that acute hyperventilation actually occurs during panic in such patients; lowered resting levels are an indication of heightened sensitivity of the blood buffer system to increases in CO_2, and predispose to acute overbreathing but are not necessarily an indication that it occurs specifically during panic attacks. That is, lowered resting level of pCO_2 itself is not accompanied by the bodily sensations associated with panic but acute hyperventilation is. This is because the sensations are induced by decreases in pH; in chronically lowered pCO_2 pH normalises, and no sensations are experienced. It is therefore necessary to demonstrate acute hyperventilation (which would produce sensations through changes in pH) in panic patients if the general model of panic is to be directly applied to hyperventilation induced sensations.

4. Effects of Stress and Panic on Respiration in Panic Patients

It is important to show that panic attack patients who recognise a strong similarity between the physical sensations associated with their panic attacks and the effects of overbreathing actually hyperventilate when in situations in which they are prone to develop panic attacks. The single case experiments described below investigate this crucially important question. Measures of pCO_2 were taken in several panic attack patients before and after they were exposed to situations in which they were prone to develop panic attacks. All of these patients were individuals who perceived a strong similarity between the effects of overbreathing and their panic attacks, and responded well to a hyperventilation based treatment.

Cases 1 and 2 (Salkovskis, Clark and Jones 1986):

Patient 1 was a 27 year old male, with a ten year history of panic attacks which occurred mostly in social situations. The most prominent symptoms he complained of were dizziness, parasthesiae, sweating, nausea and fear. When anxious he thought he might make a fool of himself, and usually left the situation as quickly as he could. He also avoided social situations wherever possible. He was treated initially using the strategy described above. When first referred, his resting pCO_2 was within the low normal range, and he was experiencing a mean of 2.6 panic attacks over the seven weeks of baseline. Treatment resulted in a reduction in panic attacks to 1 per week, but he still remained somewhat anxious in social situations. He considered that his control over his anxiety had improved, but he was still avoiding some situations because of a persistent tendency to experience unpleasant bodily sensations when called upon to talk in social settings.

Graded exposure treatment did not produce any further improvement in his report of anxiety in such situations. It was noted that, in the course of treatment sessions, this patient took frequent deep breaths and used more air than appeared to be necessary when talking normally, although he was not aware of doing this. Similar clinical observations had been made with other patients who experienced panic attacks during speech. An experiment to examine this phenomenon was therefore carried out, using the same respiratory measurement techniques described in study 2 above. The patient's resting pCO_2 was measured, then he was asked to discuss a topic he found anxiety provoking for five minutes, at which point a further pCO_2 measure was taken. Half an hour later, the procedure was repeated with a neutral topic being discussed and further measures taken. On the patient's next visit to the clinic, the whole procedure was repeated, but with the order of topics (anxiety provoking and neutral) reversed. The results (shown in Fig. 6a) indicated that, in this patient, speech is associated with a reduction in pCO_2 irrespective of topic. Treatment was specifically directed at correcting this, with the patient being taught to talk more slowly and to avoid gasping between sentences. Following a single session of such training, his pCO_2 during speech showed a drop of only 2 mm Hg.

Although the results observed with patient 1 are consistent with the hypothesis that hyperventilation occurs in situations in which he was prone to panic attacks, an alternative explanation was also possible. Perhaps reductions in pCO_2 occurred during speaking irrespective of whether giving a speech is a situation which tends to provoke a panic attack. In order to investigate this possibility, the experiment was repeat-

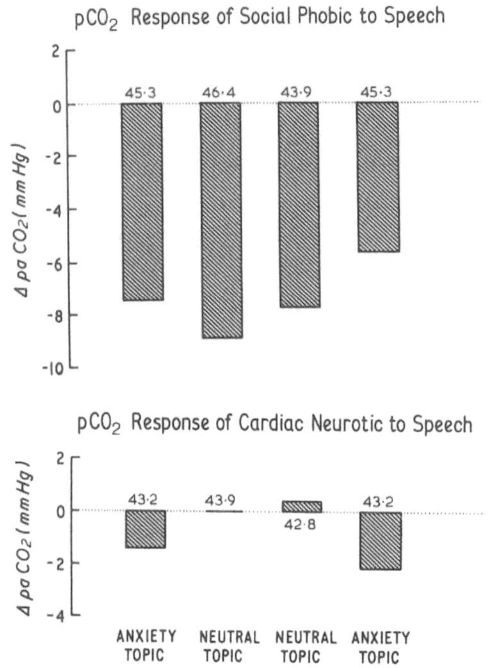

Fig. 6. Changes in pCO_2 during speech in cases 1 and 2 (figures represent resting level). (From Salkovskis, Clark and Jones 1986.)

ed with a second patient who was chosen because he showed no overlap with patient 1 in terms of situations which provoked anxiety but was similar in other respects, particularly in terms of the stage of treatment he had reached.

Patient 2 was a 35 year old male, with a 2 year history of panic attacks which could occur at any time, but which frequently followed exercise. The main symptoms he complained of were precordial pain, dizziness, feeling faint, palpitations, weak legs, palpitations and breathlessness. Thoughts accompanying his panic attacks were related to ideas of having an undetected heart condition. He was avoiding any exercise, including walking and going up stairs. Following treatment, his panic attack frequency had dropped from a mean of 11.3 per week over 5 weeks to 1.3 per week. Symptoms occurred most frequently when he noticed bodily disturbance, and he had never experienced symptoms during social interaction, which he felt distracted him from his symptoms. During the experiment the same procedures were carried out as had been used for patient 1. The effect is illustrated in Fig. 6b, which shows a slight drop in pCO_2 occurred only during discussion of his anxiety problem, in this case fear of heart disease. The magnitude of the change was small, and no change in anxiety was reported. This was to be expected, as the patient had previously indicated that simply talking about his problem did not provoke panic attacks.

From the results of patient 2, it would appear that speaking per se does not produce a marked drop in pCO_2 in panic patients. However, an additional artefactual explanation of the results observed with patient 1 could be proposed. He had been in treatment for a while before the start of the experiment and it could be argued that the things he had learned in treatment about the hypothesised relationship between overbreathing and panic allowed him to guess the experimenters expectation and either intentionally comply with the prediction, or increase his ventilation as a result of heightened awareness of his breathing. Such effects would be less likely to occur in patients who had not received the hyperventilation based treatment at the time that the experiments were conducted.

Cases 3 and 4 (Salkovskis, Clark and Jones 1986):

Two further patients were selected, and this time the experiments were conducted before treatment began. Both patients were routine psychiatric referrals, and hyperventilation had never previously been considered as a diagnosis. Patient 3, a social phobic, was selected specifically on the basis of reporting anxiety attacks occurring during social interaction, especially when she was talking. Symptoms complained of included palpitations, dizziness, feelings of faintness, sweating, feeling shaky, sweating and feeling she was going to choke. Problem duration was 2 years. Patient 4 had major fears about the possibility of having a serious heart attack and was selected on the basis of reporting cardiac symptoms being brought on by worries concerning her heart. Symptoms included chest pain and tightening, breathlessness, parasthesiae, palpitations and faintness. Duration of problem was 4 years. During three weeks of baseline, diary records showed mean panic attack frequencies of 12.7 and 17 per week respectively. Neither patient was given any indication of the importance attached to the respiratory measurements, and on debriefing both expressed surprise at the purpose of the experiment.

In each instance, the patients were subjected to the same procedure before any therapy for the panic attacks was given. During the first session, pCO_2 was measured at rest, following 5 minutes talk about the nature of their anxiety problems, at the end of 30 minutes rest and completing questionnaires, and following 5 minutes talk on topics which did not provoke anxiety. On the second occasion, similar measures were taken at rest, following 5 minutes of imagery about having cardiac symptoms, collapsing and having to be rushed to hospital, after 30 minutes of rest, and after 5 minutes of visualising a pleasant scene. The effects of these procedures on pCO_2 can be seen in Fig. 7a and 7b, together with the values for resting pCO_2. For the socially phobic patient, large decreases of pCO_2 occurred during speech and not during cardiac or pleasant imagery, whilst the cardiac neurotic patient only showed a drop in pCO_2 during cardiac imagery.

Ratings of anxiety using a 100 point visual analogue scale (VAS) were also taken. Patient 3 reported increases of greater than 30 "suds" following both periods of speech, whilst patient 4 only reported an increase of this magnitude during cardiac imagery. On each of these occasions the patients also reported some bodily symptoms characteristic of their panic attacks. Patient 4 reported that she had had a panic attack during "cardiac" imagery (although not severe enough to curtail the procedures), while patient 3 reported she knew she "would have had a proper do" if she had had to continue talking longer. Both patients responded well to the treatment, and remained free of panic attacks (as recorded on behavioural diaries) at 12 month follow-up.

Case 5 (Salkovskis, Warwick, Clark and Wessels 1986):

In the cases described above, it was possible to demonstrate substantial decreases in pCO_2 during contrived stress in situations which closely resembled the situations which usually triggered panic attacks in the patients' everyday life. Nonetheless, the stressors used were contrived situations, making generalisation to naturally occurring panic speculative. However, we were fortunate enough to be able to directly measure respiratory parameters in a further patient during naturally occurring panic attacks. Moreover, it proved possible to readily (and ethically) obtain arterial samples for the direct determination of $paCO_2$ and pH. Direct measurement of pH is particularly important because the sensations which arise from overbreathing are directly related to respiratory alkalosis (increased pH produced by lowered $paCO_2$) rather than pCO_2 changes *per se*.

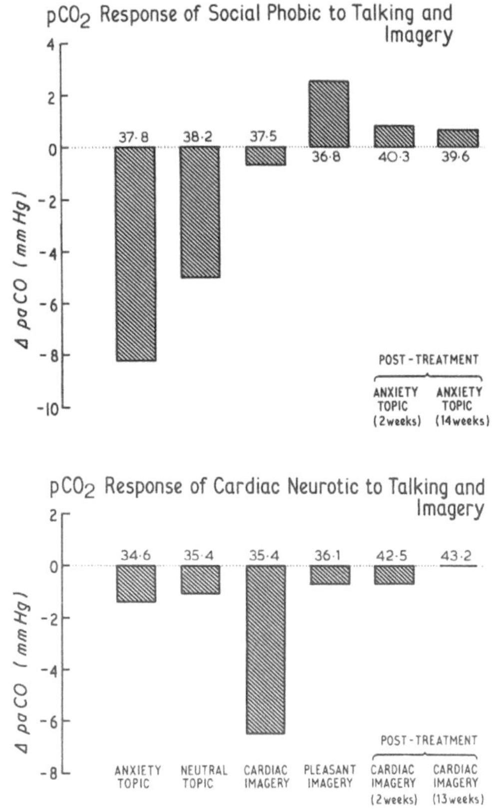

Fig. 7. Changes in pCO_2 during speech and imagery in cases 3 and 4 (figures represent resting level). (From Salkovskis, Clark and Jones 1986.)

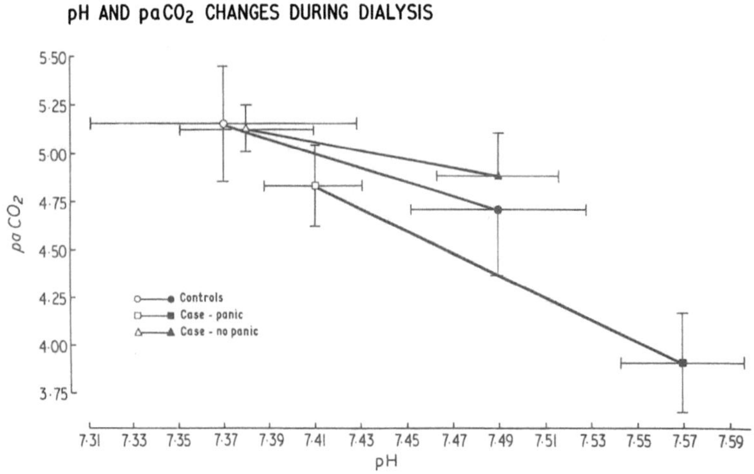

Fig. 8. $paCO_2$ (kPa) and pH at start of dialysis (open symbols) and end of dialysis (closed symbols). (Reproduced by permission from Salkovskis, Warwick, Clark and Wessels (1986) A demonstration of acute hyperventilation during naturally occurring panic attacks. Behav. Res. Ther. **24,** Pergamon Press.)

The patient, a 28 year old man, was referred because he was consistently experiencing panic towards the end of thrice-weekly acetate-buffered haemodialysis sessions. He had been undergoing dialysis for acute on chronic renal failure for seven years. Panic attacks had started six months prior to referral, and proved resistant to available interventions, such as parenteral benzodiazepines and supportive psychotherapy.

Assessment on referral suggested that the panic attacks which occurred at the end of dialysis were triggered by the bodily sensations and increased respiration induced by the metabolic changes associated with acetate buffered haemodialysis. Renal patients normally attribute these sensations to the normal process of dialysis because of their clear temporal link with the procedures; however, in this particular instance, the patient's previous experience of the association between sensations of the intensity and nature he was experiencing and severe life-threatening complications led him to conclude "these sensations indicate that dialysis itself is about to kill me". This worrying thought was associated with further increases in respiration, which added to the alkalosis from which the sensations had originated in the first instance. Analysis of arterial blood samples (which are easily taken during dialysis) indicated that, during panic attacks, $paCO_2$ dropped and pH increased by greater amounts and to more extreme levels than observed at times when panic was not experienced, or in control dialysis patients, as shown in Fig. 8.

Deliberate overbreathing away from the dialysis machine exactly reproduced the symptoms the patient reported during panic attacks. This demonstration was used as the basis for reattribution of the sensations onto stress induced hyperventilation and treatment along the lines already described above. This intervention proved highly successful, and the patient remained panic free up to 1 year follow up.

5. Discussion

The treatment studies provide encouraging support for the view that an intervention directed at the re-attribution of sensations away from catastrophic interpretations and to the effects of stress induced hyperventilation is effective as a treatment for panic attacks. Substantial changes in panic frequency and severity were demonstrated in a period shorter than a stable baseline, ruling out the possibility that spontaneous remission was responsible for the results obtained. The evidence is also consistent with the view that initial improvement was not brought about by increased exposure to previously avoided situations. It seems most likely that there are a number of effective components in the intervention package; in particular the extremely rapid initial reduction in panic attack frequency and self reported anxiety in the Behaviour Test might suggest that the cognitive element (reattribution of the panic attacks to a less threatening cause and development of more adaptive reactions to physiological arousal) may have had considerable impact. This is certainly consistent with previous clinical reports that simply identifying the nature of the attacks through a provocation test (brief forced ventilation) is often enough to produce a complete remission of attacks, particularly in cases with a recent onset of attacks (Lum 1976). The success of efforts at controlling panic attacks by respiratory and cognitive manoeuvres was utilised here to enhance such effects by the repeated presentation of information which was consonant with non-catastrophic interpretations of bodily sensations, and highly dissonant with the patients previous catastrophic attributions.

That respiratory training and a consequent enhanced control of bodily symptoms could be actively involved is consistent with the pCO_2 changes observed in the course of treatment. An overall decrease in sensitivity (increased threshold) to respiratory challenge would be expected to result from this change. That exposure may be involved in another sense is also possible, as the training included repeatedly overbreathing then controlling the symptoms thus experienced. Such a procedure, as well as improving respiratory self-control, has the effect of repeatedly exposing the patient to the feared (and avoided) physiological symptoms of panic, and could be expected to produce a reduction in the cognitive response to these.

The second set of studies show that, in some patients, the respiratory response to panic-related situations is sufficiently large to provide a physical trigger for the hypothesised mis-attribution. At the very least, the magnitude of pCO_2 change demonstrated in these patients will readily produce the range of somatic symptoms associated with respiratory alkalosis. It is therefore clear that during the time in which respiration was monitored, patients will have experienced the physical symptoms which accompany acute changes in $paCO_2$ and pH. Furthermore, all of these patients showed most of the physical symptoms of their panic attacks within 45 seconds of forced ventilation during a provocation test, although none had previously attributed their symptoms to hyperventilation.

6. Conclusions

The work described here is encouraging because, within the design constraints of the outcome studies, it was possible to establish that a treatment derived from the cognitive model is effective with patients in whom there is other evidence to suggest that hyperventilation may be involved in their panic attacks. Other evidence supporting the application of this model to panic attacks in such patients lies in (i) the chronically low resting pCO_2 levels in panic patients compared to matched controls; (ii) the recognition by most panic patients in the treatment studies of strong similarity between sensations experienced during panic attacks and the effects of a period of brief voluntary hyperventilation; (iii) the close relationship between treatment outcome and the perception of such similarity; (iv) the demonstration that some panic patients acutely hyperventilate under stress and during panic to a degree which will produce many bodily sensations (even although they have no awareness of this increased respiration).

That hyperventilation alone cannot account for panic attacks is evident from the individual difference studies (Clark and

Hemsley 1982; Svebak and Grossman 1985) and from the general observation that hyperventilation *per se* (however prolonged or acute) does not generally result in panic attacks. Even in panic patients in whom hyperventilation is strongly implicated, overbreathing does not invariably produce panic; indeed, as treatment progresses, repeated deliberate overbreathing can be observed to result in substantial decrements in subjective appraisal of anxiety without any comparable decline in bodily sensations experienced (c.f. the effects of repeated induction of symptoms by CO_2 inhalation reported by van den Hout and Griez 1984).

Further evaluation of the model requires the demonstration that panic patients are more likely to catastrophically misinterpret bodily sensations than others; a more direct demonstration of the role of cognitions in mediating the affective response to bodily sensations, and an analysis of the effective elements in the respiratory control treatment. The advantage of a hyperventilation-based cognitive treatment lies in its relative simplicity and brevity as compared to conventional cognitive therapy for anxiety (c.f. Beck, Emery and Greenberg 1985). It is encouraging to note that 60% of panic patients recognise a strong similarity between the sensations produced by voluntary hyperventilation and symptoms of naturally occurring panic attacks. This indicates that this treatment may be applicable to a substantial proportion of panic patients. There is also some evidence that similar processes may be involved in other patient groups, such as unexplained chest pain with disproportionate breathlessness (Bass, Cawley, Wade, Ryan, Gardener, Hutchinson and Jackson 1983; see also case 4 above). Further developments in this area are therefore likely to be of benefit to a considerable number of patients.

7. References

American Psychiatric Association (1980) Diagnostic and Statistical Manual of Mental Disorders, Third Edition. American Psychiatric Association, Washington

Balke B, Ellis JP, Wells JG (1958) Adaptive responses to hyperventilation. J Appl Physiol 12:269–277

Bass C, Cawley R, Wade C, Ryan KC, Gardener WN, Hutchinson DCS, Jackson G (1983) Unexplained breathlessness and psychiatric morbidity in patients with normal and abnormal coronary arteries. The Lancet, i, 605–609

Beck AT, Beamsderfer A (1974) Assessment of depression: the depression inventory. In: Pichot P (ed) Modern problems in pharmacopsychiatry. (Vol 7) Karger, Basel

Beck AT, Emery G, Greenberg RL (1985) Anxiety disorders and phobias: A cognitive perspective. Basic Books, New York

Beck AT, Laude R, Bohnert M (1974) Ideational components of anxiety neurosis. Arch Gen Psychiatry 3:319–325

Cambell EJM, Howell JBL (1962) Measurement of mixed venous pCO_2. Brit Med J ii:630–633

Clark DM (1979) Therapeutic aspects of increasing pCO_2 by behavioural means. Unpublished M. Phil. thesis, University of London

Clark DM (1986) A cognitive approach to panic. Beh Res Ther, in press

Clark DM, Hemsley DR (1982) Effects of hyperventilation: individual variability and its relation to personality. J Beh Ther Exp Psychiatry 13:41–47

Clark DM, Salkovskis PM, Chalkley AJ (1985) Respiratory control as a treatment for panic attacks. J Beh Ther Exp Psychiatry 16:23–30

Gibson HB (1978) A form of behaviour therapy for some states diagnosed as "affective disorder". Beh Res Ther 16:191–195

Goldstein AJ, Chambless DL (1978) A re-analysis of agoraphobia. Behav Ther 9:47–59

Hibbert GA (1984) Ideational components of anxiety: their origin and content. Br J Psychiatry 144:618–624

Huey SR, West SG (1983) Hyperventilation: Its relation to symptom experience and anxiety. J Abnorm Psychol 92:422–432

Kerr WJ, Dalton JW, Gliebe PA (1937) Some physical phenomena associated with anxiety states and their relation to hyperventilation. Ann Intern Med 11:961–992

Keselman HJ, Rogan JC (1980) Repeated measures F tests and psychophysiological research: Controlling the number of false positives. Psychophysiology 17:499–503

Lang PJ (1970) Stimulus control, response control and the desensitization of fear. In: Levis DJ (ed) Learning approaches to therapeutic behavior. Aldine Press, Chicago

Lum LC (1976) The syndrome of habitual chronic hyperventilation. Hill OW (ed) Modern trends in psychosomatic medicine. 3, Butterworths, London

Marks IM, Mathews A (1979) Brief standard self-rating for phobic patients. Beh Res Ther 17:263–267

Salkovskis PM, Jones DRO, Clark DM (1986) Respiratory Control in the treatment of panic attacks: replication and extension with concurrent measures of behaviour and pCO_2. Br J Psychiatry, in press

Salkovskis PM, Clark DM, Jones DRO (1986) A Psychosomatic mechanism in anxiety attacks; the role of hyperventilation in social anxiety and cardiac neurosis. In: Lacey H, Sturgeon J (eds) Proceedings of the 15th European Conference on Psychosomatic Research, London 1984

Salkovskis PM, Warwick HMC, Clark DM, Wessels DJ (1986) A demonstration of acute hyperventilation during naturally occurring panic attacks. Beh Res Ther 24:91–94

Schachter S, Singer JE (1962) Cognitive, social and physiological determinants of emotional state. Psychol Rev 69:379–399

Seuss WM, Alexander AB, Smith DD, Sweeney HW, Marion RJ (1980) The effects of psychological stress on respiration: a preliminary study of anxiety and hyperventilation. Psychophysiology 17:535–540

Stampler FM (1982) Panic disorder: description, conceptualisation, and implications for treatment. Clin Psychol Review 2:469–486

Svebak S, Grossman P (1985) How aversive is hyperventilation? Clinical Respiratory Physiology, 21, in press

van den Hout MA, Griez E (1984) Carbondioxide and anxiety: an experimental approach to a clinical claim. Thesis, Rijksuniversiteit Maastricht

11. Exposure In-Vivo with Panic Management for Agoraphobia: Treatment Rationale and Longterm Outcome

Iver Hand, Jörg Angenendt, Martina Fischer, and Cornelia Wilke

1. Introduction

During the 1970's a series of international treatment studies, pioneered and led by British groups from London and Oxford, seemed to have established some of the best documented and validated, highly specific short-term treatments for a rather chronic illness in the whole field of psychotherapy research: exposure in-vivo for agoraphobia. Since the beginning of this decade, parallel to the introduction of DSM-III, an increasing amount of basic research and clinical studies on panic disorder, panic attacks and agoraphobia with panic attacks seems to question this empirical and experimental knowledge.

In this paper, we shall present data from a multivariate, long-term prospective and retrospective follow-up study with agoraphobics after short-term exposure treatment. This is the first study to compare directly immediate and long-term effects of the three most popular modes of exposure in vivo: individual and group exposure (therapist aided) and Home Based Treatment (HBT; manual aided). This is also the first follow-up study with agoraphobics to simultaneously investigate: comparative outcomes in mild and severe, mono- and multisymptomatically disturbed agoraphobics; comparative assessment of "gainers" and "losers" from treatment, as well as their "multisymptomatic development" during treatment and follow-up.

All self-rating scales were used before and during treatment as well as throughout all follow-up assessments (prospective part of the study). At their last follow-up, patients also received a detailed, structured interview for current and retrospective evaluation.

Most patients had received psycho-pharmacological treatment before exposure and were taken off such medication before exposure started.

This study supplements a series of previous follow-up investigations with agoraphobics that have set standards in psychotherapy research: Marks 1971; Emmelkamp and Kuipers 1979; McPherson et al. 1980; Munby and Johnston 1980; Cohen et al. 1984.

Although these studies show vast differences in kind and extent of treatment procedures, assessment instruments, criteria of success, and length of follow-up they agreed to the following: two thirds to three fourths of the patients showed clinically relevant and statistically significant reductions of their phobic avoidance and complaints; positive changes tended to generalize to other neurotic complaints (the mostly assessed variable being depression); personal and social functioning of two thirds of these patients improved enduringly; interference of phobia with daily life and professional activities was clearly reduced. Nevertheless, all these studies also indicated that at least 25% to 33% of the patients treated did not improve. Also, some shortcomings of previous follow-ups, that limit their generalizability, need to be mentioned: the study by McPherson et al. included only those patients who had improved after treatment and of those only 69% participated in follow-up; the Emmelkamp and Kuipers study relied entirely on postal follow-ups with clinical self-rating scales; the Cohen et al. study did not report effects of therapy on daily life and professional activities. Nevertheless, all studies with exposure for agoraphobia and with long-term follow-up are models for psychotherapy research: 1. a highly specific, short-term treatment is applied to a rather chronic disorder, and 2. changes are assessed over longer periods of time. By this, clear conclusions can be reached regarding specific treatment effects as opposed to changes due to other life events (Lambert and Bergin 1978; Agras and Berkowitz 1980; Barlow and Wolfe 1981). Even in behavior therapy, such studies made up 1% of the articles published until 1979 (Agras and Berkowitz 1980).

Before we present the results of our study, our exposure concept will be described in some detail, as it may make some of our results more understandable.

2. Experimental Design

From 1976 to 1983 some 250 agoraphobic patients received intake interviews in our unit. The demand for treatment by far exceeded this number.

In 1984, we started a 1–8 year follow-up (FU) study with these patients. For methodological reasons patients had to be split into two groups: study I, 1–4 years (1980–1983) and study II, 5–8 years (1976–1979) after treatment. In 1980 we had introduced a new set of self-rating scales for neurotic multisymptomatology (c.f. Hand and Zaworka 1982), which since has been given to all our patients throughout treatment and follow-up. Here, we shall report the data from the first group (study I).

Main aims of both studies are: 1. multivariate assessment of the long-term "field efficacy" (Agras and Berkowitz 1980) of a short and highly specific treatment, and 2. comparison of patients who were improved in their phobia at FU (gainers) with those who were not (losers) to identify reasons for and consequences of "failures in behavior therapy" (cf. Foa and Emmelkamp 1983).

This study is a combination of a **prospective** (data from symptom self-rating scales) and a **retrospective** (data from a structured interview) follow-up.

2.1. Treatments: Exposure In-Vivo and Panic Management

Patients received one of the following modes of exposure in-vivo as their main and usually only intervention: individual exposure; group exposure; Home Based Treatment (HBT). Therapist-aided exposure (first two modes) was conducted according to the exposure-panic management concept developed by Hand et al. (1974). It is applied within three to five treatment days over one or two weeks, respectively. For HBT we used our authorized German translations (publication in preparation) of the manuals for patient, spouse and therapist, developed by Matthews et al. (1977, 1981). HBT patients had five brief contacts with the therapist in his office over a period of four weeks.

Over the past ten years, *exposure in-vivo* has been recognized as the most effective single treatment intervention in clinically relevant phobias, particularly in agoraphobia (detailed reviews in Marks 1975; Mathews et al. 1981; Chambless and Goldstein 1982; Thorpe and Burns 1983; Thorpe et al. 1984). Early warnings about potential dangers of exposure in-vivo arose from misunderstandings or misapplications of this treatment technique. Shipley and Boudewyns (1980), in an international survey which comprised some 3500 patients, could demonstrate that harmful effects are extremely rare events. More recent publications on the importance of antidepressant medication as an essential, additional treatment to exposure in-vivo, or even as the single most effective treatment for "agoraphobia with panic attacks" (Sheehan et al. 1980; Zitrin et al. 1980; Klein 1981; Mavissakalian et al. 1983), as yet have not proven their claims. They show a tendency to dismiss well established results from behavior therapy. Also, these studies do not constitute comparisons of proper exposure in-vivo versus medication. With their generalized claims with regard to their panic model and its therapeutic consequences, they may turn out more clinically misleading than stimulating (cf. Marks 1983; Hand 1984; intense controversial discussions of this issue in Archives of General Psychiatry since 1983).

Group exposure in-vivo probably has become the most widely used therapist-aided application of exposure for agoraphobics. Yet, important elements of the original mode by Hand et al. (1974) seem to have been omitted in some of the subsequent studies. As they remained essential in the Hamburg study – which includes a long-term, multiple replication of the 1974 Maudsley study – they are to be emphasized again:
a. Panic (peak anxiety) management; b. Depression and "emotional distress" management; c. High group cohesion for mutual support and motivation.

a. Panic management: is the second (to behavioral exposure itself) most important element in this treatment concept. Therefore, patients are taken off psychotropic medication for at least one week before exposure – even if this induces withdrawal symptoms from previous tranquilizer medication. Ideally, patients are to experience exposure under difficult environmental and emotional conditions, in order to rebuild lasting self-confidence. Patients should not experience in-vivo sessions as easier than phobic daily life conditions – otherwise they would maintain the phobic anticipatory anxiety of not being able to cope "when it really comes to the worst". In particular, patients who had panic attacks in and outside phobic situations prior to treatment are to experience those as early in exposure as possible ("exposure proper" for agoraphobia with panic attacks). The therapist takes care, that his "prescription" of panic does not have the reverse effect in the sense of a paradoxical intervention.

Confrontation even with the most feared situations is tried already on the first treatment day. Experience of peak anxiety (panic) usually lasts for some to ten, rarely up to twenty minutes. As soon as patients report a definite decline of high or peak anxiety in the same situation that seemed to have raised it, the next phobic situation is entered. The criterion for moving is the patient's experience-induced new cognitive response: "I can cope." Instructions during exposure are simple, though difficult to follow at the beginning: "Allow all your feelings to grow; observe and describe to yourself the reality of your surroundings and the sensations of your body; do neither phantasize your phobic phantasies, nor try to suppress anxiety or other unpleasant feelings by mental or motor avoidance manoeuvers; try to give yourself always another ten seconds to tolerate the situation or your own, almost unbearable responses to it."

Under those conditions, which may lead to a "corrective emotional experience", most patients develop their own "cognitive restructuring" with regard to the phobic situation and their responses to it. Obviously, this approach works best with those patients who have experienced panic in the past and are lucky to experience it early during exposure. In groups, these patients are the most convincing models for their peers.

So far, there are no publications that convincingly reveal an impact of the level of "anxiety during exposure" upon outcome of treatment. But, the usual procedure of computing mean anxiety levels over hours of exposure seems bound to hide relevant information. In our unit, Priebe (1980) found that agoraphobics who had repeatedly experienced high "fluctuations of anxiety" (i.e. rapid decreases of acute peak anxiety states) during treatment did best at the end of treatment and in short-term follow-up. They did not necessarily have the highest mean anxiety ratings over a whole exposure session. This result seems to confirm the clinical impressions described, e.g. in the 1974 Maudsley study.

b. Depression and "emotional distress" management is conducted the same way. Agoraphobics frequently complain about intermittent states of severe depression, which may be closely linked to feelings of insufficiency and lowered self-esteem resulting from humiliating experiences as a phobic.

But, depression can also follow the experience of success, e.g. in exposure treatment. After the usual experience of impressive decreases of phobic anxiety during the first treatment day, patients often go home in an elevated, almost hypo-manic mood. But, in the following night they tend to have nightmares – experiencing in their dreams all those disasters that did not occur during exposure. Typically, when the second exposure session is due (by design) one day later, they come depressed and almost too scared to be daring again. This state of mood and mind is "re-labeled" by the therapist: the bad mood and low spirit being interpreted as a unique chance for the patient to experience in subsequent exposure this very day that coping with anxiety and depression is possible, and that this experience by itself might become the optimal antidepressant. And this is what actually happens to the "gainers" in treatment.

We never raise the expectation that treatment will completely eliminate episodes of anxiety or depression. Instead, we want to provide the real-life experience that the consequences of "giving in" to those feelings on a motor-behavior level probably create to a large extent the "illness" of chronic agoraphobia. If disconnected from phobic anticipatory cognition (with low self-esteem), the occurrence of further anxiety attacks and depressive episodes will, for the majority of patients, be rare and usually manageable events.

c. High group cohesion: was tried to be achieved in all our groups, following the procedure described for the highly cohesive groups in the Maudsley study. High cohesion probably is the single most powerful motivational variable for cooperation in exposure in-vivo (cf. Hafner and Marks 1976).

Some additional, important aspects of this exposure concept are:

– Intermittent escape is allowed in our approach, though never encouraged. It appears important not to threaten a patient's autonomy by contracts in which he subscribes himself to "being held" in the phobic situation if he cannot manage to do so by himself. Some treatment centers seem to apply much more direct external control, and patients not infrequently seem to expect, and to be afraid of, such a therapist attitude. Though this attitude may seem plausible from learning theory concepts, it appears rather dangerous from an interactional point of view. Therefore, when intermittent avoidance occurs, we try to reassess motivation for change (in phobic as well as in daily life activities) with the patient – and this usually leads to the patient's decision to enter the situation again at his own will.

– During the three to five treatment days patients are to learn to believe in their coping ability with peak anxiety and other unpleasant emotions and bodily sensations – rather than to expect to become immediately free of it. The latter is rather to be expected from long-term, continued self-exposure and increasing alternative behavior after treatment. Treatment is interpreted as a brief challenge to a stereotyped phobic self-concept and way of life – and it is tried to convince the patient that it is his choice what to make of it.

– This exposure concept emphasizes the main role of exposure of the patient to his own responses, rather than to the phobic trigger situation. *The experience of panic in a phobic trigger situation is mainly used to teach management of panic rather than tolerance of the trigger situation.* With such a concept, it becomes less important whether panic attacks do occur only in phobic situations or "anywhere". One also has to consider that quite some "spontaneous" panic attacks may result from cognitive anticipatory exposure to phobic situations, not always detected in the clinical interviews. To give an example of exposure to the own response: a thunderstorm phobic was treated by inducing his main phobic complaint, severe dizziness, in the treatment office and by teaching him coping responses; subsequently he was able to expose himself to the next real thunderstorm without any major problems. Even extreme physiological panic responses can be modified with this concept in one treatment session, like, e.g. fainting in a blood phobic, with twenty seconds of "silence" in his electrocardiogram (Hand and Schroeder 1980).

– In quite some patients, high emotional arousal during exposure spontaneously leads to continued behavioral (self-)analysis of previously not available information; it may thus extend the areas of intervention (Hand 1986).

For Thorpe et al. (1984) this group exposure concept, published in 1974, seems very similar to contemporary cognitive-behavioral procedures. In particular, they see these similarities to Bandura's (1978) concept of self-efficacy, with the notion that confidence rather than fear is modified in effective treatment. The "behavioral panic management" in group exposure in-vivo also seems to be in accordance with latest developments in "cognitive" psychology, which recently has come to favor a "motor theory" of cognition again (Mahoney 1983).

The panic management element in *group exposure* was applied to the *individual exposure* in our trial as well. In contrast, there are quite a few major differences in the coping concept used in HBT. This does not deliberately induce peak anxiety or panic. Rather, it encourages avoidance of intense emotional states, as the patient applies exposure either alone or with the help of his spouse. Speed of exposure is left entirely to the patient, as is the choice of distance from home for self-exposure. Thus, within the first few weeks or months after treatment, patients with therapist-aided exposure generally have done far more exercises further away from their homes than patients in HBT. We shall see later how this affects immediate and long-term outcome.

2.2. Patients

Criteria for diagnosing "agoraphobia" were much the same as in the British studies (cf. Marks 1970). The majority of our patients would also have been diagnosed as "agoraphobics with panic attacks" according to DSM-III. We diagnose a patient "agoraphobic" and appoint him to the respective treatment, regardless of sub-symptomatology like hyperventilation, tachycardia, severe perspiration or the expectation of fainting or going crazy. Provided these sub-symptoms are clearly secondary to the typical agoraphobic behaviors and cognitions, this symptomatology will also be secondary in exposure treatment.

"Cardiac phobia" would be regarded a sub-symptom of agoraphobia, if it mainly existed in connection with agoraphobic situations. On the other hand, we would give the main diagnosis of "cardiac phobia" in a patient who is primarily worried about the health of his heart, even if one possible secondary consequence of this would be severely restricted outdoor living (secondary agoraphobia). This patient would in many aspects receive quite a different treatment from that of an agoraphobic. With this kind of diagnosing, it

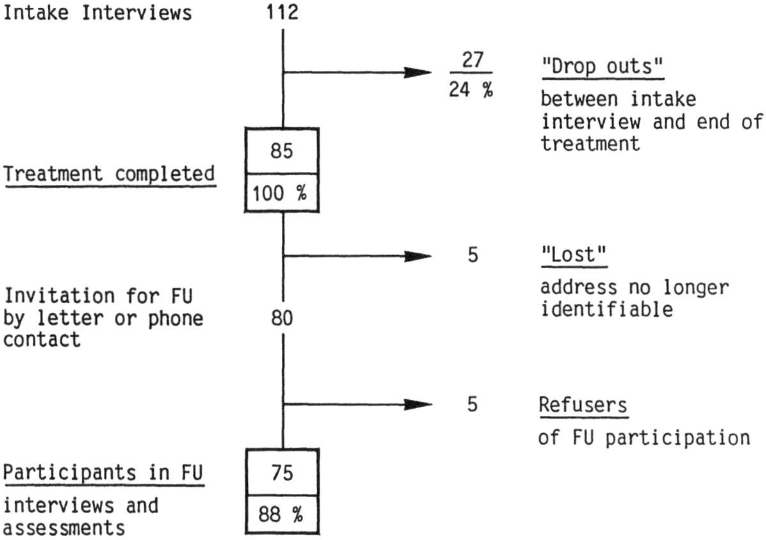

Table. 1. Agoraphobic patients in the Hamburg Behavior Therapy outpatient unit 1980–1983

turns out that the vast majority of "cardiac phobics" in our unit are male, whereas the vast majority of agoraphobics are female.

From 1980–1983 we conducted altogether 112 intake interviews with agoraphobic patients.

Table 1 shows that of these 112 patients, 27 (24%) did not participate in, or complete, treatment. A similar "drop-out" rate has been reported from other centers. It comprises very heterogeneous subgroups – including those who: a. successfully applied exposure by themselves after having been explained the principle in the intake interview (cf. Hand et al. 1974); b. found other therapists while on our waiting list (of 3–12 months!); c. dropped out of exposure treatment. A separate follow-up of all these patients is currently under way.

Of the 85 patients who had completed treatment, five could not be located any more, and another five were unwilling to participate in FU. With 88% of the treated patients participating in the interviews and test assessments, results can be regarded as fairly representative for the whole sample treated.

The 75 FU participants are to be devided into four subsamples with regard to *length of follow-up:* $\leqq 18$ months, n = 12 (16%); $\leqq 30$ months, n = 31 (41%); $\leqq 42$ months, n = 16 (21%); > 42 months, n = 16 (21%). Thus, 83% had a follow-up of more than 1.5 years, including the 42% with more than 2.5 years. Length of FU did not affect outcome. Patients' demographic data are summarized in Table 2.

The vast majority of patients were female, living with a spouse, around 32 years old, agoraphobic for about 6.5 years, and 95% had sought professional help prior to behavior therapy. About half of them were working outside their family.

2.3. Assessments

A battery of self-rating instruments was employed in order to simultaneously assess the presence and the *development over time* of a variety of neurotic symptoms. This seemed necessary, as agoraphobics – like other more severely disturbed neurotics – frequently suffer from severe multisymptomatology (cf. Chambless and Goldstein 1982; Thorpe and Burns 1983). A new methodological approach for this kind of "time-dynamic" assessment has been proposed by Hand and Zaworka (1982).

The following self-rating scales were used:

Main phobia: Fear Survey Schedule, FSS (Hallam and Hafner 1978), subscale agoraphobia. "Behavioral Resistance Scale", BRS, a 99 mm visual analog scale, devel-

Table 2. Demographic data

No. of cases	75		
Sex:			
Female	63 (84%)		
Male	12 (16%)		
Age	x̄ = 32.40	(s = 8.24; range 18–54)	
Symptom duration	x̄ = 6.76	(s = 5.14; range 1–19)	
Years from onset of illnes to first therapist contact	x̄ = 4.33	(s = 4.06; range 0–19)	
Treatment prior to exposure	71 (95%)		
Occupational status:		Marital status:	
Work outside family	42 (56%)	With spouse	59 (79%)
House-wife/man	19 (25%)	Without spouse	16 (21%)
Unemployed	10 (13%)		
Sick leave/pens.	2 (3%)		
Missing data	2 (3%)		

oped in our unit to assess the extent to which a person is able to continue "alternative motor behavior" in spite of cognitive-emotional phobic reactions. This is the reverse formulation of behavioral avoidance to indicate the degree of motivation to resist or to overcome phobic impulses. Finally, patients' subjective estimate of symptom interference with daily life activities is assessed on a similar 99 mm scale. We did not use a behavioral avoidance test, as this does not seem to give very reliable information about the actual avoidance in daily life (Hand et al. 1974).

Other phobias: FSS-subscale social anxiety and FSS-total phobia score, including animal, blood-injury and other specific phobias.

Other symptoms: Depression scale, DS, by v. Zerssen (1976), which correlates 0.8 with the British Wakefield scale; Hamburger Zwangs-Inventar, HZI, for obsessions and compulsions (Zaworka et al. 1983; English translation available from the authors); scale I, functional somatic complaints, of the Freiburger Persönlichkeitsinventar, FPI-A (Fahrenberg et al. 1973, 1984) – this trait-scale has a 0.75 correlation with a state-scale on functional somatic complaints, consisting of 78 items (Freiburger Beschwerdeliste, FBL by Fahrenberg 1975). Criteria for selection of these scales are described in Hand and Zaworka (1982).

Trait scales: Freiburger Persönlichkeitsinventar (s. above). In all subsequent tables, symptom ratings will be shown in this sequence.

Assessment intervals: Assessments were made *pre-treatment (T1), post-treatment (T2), 6-months (T3) and long-term FU (T4).* Patients had advance knowledge of the follow-ups.

An additional structured FU interview was developed and applied by two of the authors (Angenendt and Fischer), who had had no prior contact to the patients. The following areas were covered:

Symptom-related variables: The Marks and Watson (1971) Scales on Phobic Anxiety and Avoidance were used as a structured interview, emphasizing the semantic "meaning" of each point on the 0–8 scales.

Symptom development after treatment: was indirectly assessed by the examination of additional treatments, psychotropic medication, relapses, development of additional complaints ("symptom substitution"), and of the impact of life-events upon symptom development.

Daily-life activities: Again the Marks and Watson Scales were used as a structured interview for interference of symptomatology with daily-life activities: marital and family relations; housework; occupation; leisure activities; social contacts; psychological well-being.

Retrospective evaluation of treatment by patients: comprised their causal attribution of symptom change, their experience of the therapeutic relationship, and negative experiences during or immediately after treatment. It was also tried to get patients' suggestions for changes in, or improvement of, treatment.

Data analysis: *The statistical methods* applied for data analysis will be mentioned with each step of the data presentation.

3. Results

3.1. Outcome for Total Patient Sample

3.1.1. Symptom Scales: Prospective Follow-Up

For the total patient sample (n=75), all symptom ratings on each occasion (T1–T4) are summarized by the group means (x), standard deviation (s) and the number of patients who completed the ratings (Table 3).

Better than curves or histograms, the layout of significance levels for symptom changes during treatment and follow-up intervals allows a quick assessment of relevant treatment effects as well as time-dependency of changes in different symptoms (Table 4).

Results in Tables 3 and 4 suggest the following treatment effects over time on multisymptomatic disturbance: MANOVA (Nie et al. 1980) with repeated measures on one variable reveals highly significant (SSS) changes on all variables between T1 and T4. T-tests for dependent samples for the treatment and the follow-up phase separately show clear differences in the time sequences of changes for different groups of variables. Treatment induces highly significant changes on all variables, whereas in the follow-up phase we find further significant (s) and very significant (ss) improvements only in those symptoms that were not directly tackled in treatment (cf. discussion). But, results with the gainers alone

Table 3. Symptom development over time: total sample (n=75)

Symptoms	Pre-treatment (T1)			Post-treatment (T2)			6-month FU (T3)			Last FU (T4)		
	x̄	(s)	N	x̄	(s)	N	x̄	(s)	N	x̄	(s)	N
Agoraphobia												
Agoraphobia	23.03	(6.66)	73	15.24	(7.95)	68	14.54	(7.47)	57	13.76	(8.63)	72
Behavioral resistance	40.03	(28.53)	72	65.82	(22.16)	65	69.44	(21.61)	57	68.03	(26.19)	72
Interference	67.58	(21.44)	72	43.83	(26.38)	65	34.23	(26.02)	57	36.50	(28.56)	72
Other phobias												
Social anxiety	8.86	(4.79)	73	7.47	(5.10)	68	7.25	(4.25)	56	6.43	(4.82)	72
Phobias – total score	59.67	(18.02)	73	46.97	(20.69)	68	45.67	(20.33)	57	41.49	(21.10)	72
Other symptoms												
Depression	19.89	(9.43)	72	14.59	(8.56)	69	13.98	(9.78)	57	11.35	(9.32)	72
Obsessions-compulsions	3.07	(1.76)	72	2.38	(1.71)	68	2.23	(1.66)	57	2.00	(1.52)	64
Functional somatic complaints	7.22	(1.76)	73	6.62	(2.00)	69	6.39	(1.98)	56	6.00	(2.19)	70

Table 4. Symptom development over time: when does improvement occur? Total sample (n=75)

Symptoms	Manova*:			T-test**:					
	Mean effect time			Intervention phase T1–T2			Follow-up-phase T2–T4		
	F	p	sig	T	p	sig	T	p	sig
Agoraphobia									
Agoraphobia	29.02	0.000	sss	9.46	0.000	sss	1.56	0.124	ns
Behavioral resistance	14.06	0.000	sss	-6.55	0.000	sss	-0.93	0.355	ns
Interference	28.61	0.000	sss	7.29	0.000	sss	1.97	0.053	ns
Other phobias									
Social anxiety	9.78	0.000	sss	2.95	0.004	ss	2.01	0.048	s
Phobias – total score	22.05	0.000	sss	7.18	0.000	sss	2.31	0.024	s
Other symptoms									
Depression	16.21	0.000	sss	6.15	0.000	sss	2.81	0.007	ss
Obsessions-compulsions	10.81	0.000	sss	4.65	0.000	sss	2.69	0.009	ss
Functional somatic complaints	10.42	0.000	sss	5.23	0.000	sss	2.94	0.005	ss

ns≈$p>0.05$; s≈$p\leqq 0.05$; ss≈$p\leqq 0.01$; sss≈$p\leqq 0.001$

* Results of analyses of variances for repeated measurements

** Results of T-tests for dependent samples

are quite different (3.3.2.). It is important to note that at pre-treatment on the individual level there is no straight correlation between level of phobic anxiety and degree of behavioral resistance (avoidance): Pearson's r=0.15.

3.1.2. Interview Data: Retrospective Follow-Up

Changes in phobic anxiety:
At follow-up, 33 (44%) patients rated *no or low* anxiety (0–2), 23 (31%) *slight to medium* anxiety (3–5) and 19 (25%) *severe* anxiety to panic (6–8).

The total phobia score from the assessors Marks/Watson interview correlates 0.8 with patient's self-rating on FSS-agoraphobia.

At follow-up, still 30% of the total sample experience medium (four patients of the slight to medium group scored 5) to severe anxiety in agoraphobic situations. This corresponds with the fairly high group mean of 14 on the FSS-agoraphobia scale (Table 3) at last follow-up, which is probably due to much higher ratings of these 30% of the total sample, with gainers then showing much lower means (cf. 3.3.2).

Changes in interference of phobic symptomatology with daily life activities: reveal a similar outcome to that on phobic anxiety (Table 5).

Before treatment, by far the highest interferences of agoraphobia had occurred in psychological well-being, and in occupational and leisure activities. In all areas of daily life there is a strong reduction in the percentage of patients that experience a severe degree of interference, paralleled by a strong increase of those who experience none or low interference. Results, however have to be interpreted with caution, as the "pre-treatment" scores are derived from patients' retrospective assessments. Assessors' ratings of phobic interference correlate 0.82 (Pearson's r) with patients' FSS-agoraphobia ratings at follow-up – i.e. losers experiencing persistent high phobic anxiety are also severely restricted with regard to everyday functioning.

Additional treatments during follow-up:
Treatments during follow-up may be regarded as indicaters of further subjective

Table 5. Interference of agoraphobia with daily life activities (Structured interview with Marks/Watson scale)

Daily life activities	Degree of interference 0–2 = none or low 3–5 = slight to medium 6–8 = severe	Percentage of patients Pre-treatment (retrospective evaluation!) %	Last FU %
	x̄ / (s)	3.42 / (3.10)	1.53 / (2.05)
Marital relations	None or low	45	76
	Medium	23	18
	Severe	32	6
	x̄ / (s)	3.27 / (3.06)	1.14 / (1.73)
Family relations	None or low	48	81
	Medium	18	15
	Severe	34	4
	x̄ / (s)	6.06 / (2.53)	2.41 / (2.81)
Occupation	None or low	12	62
	Medium	14	18
	Severe	74	20
	x̄ / (s)	2.72 / (2.83)	0.61 / (1.14)
Housework	None or low	55	96
	Medium	18	3
	Severe	27	1
	x̄ / (s)	5.85 / (2.45)	2.45 / (2.56)
Leisure activities	None or low	12	55
	Medium	16	26
	Severe	72	19
	x̄ / (s)	4.40 / (2.97)	1.38 / (2.17)
Social contacts	None or low	29	80
	Medium	28	12
	Severe	43	8
	x̄ / (s)	6.75 / (1.88)	2.63 / (2.49)
Psychological well-being	None or low	3	51
	Medium	18	33
	Severe	79	16
Total	x̄ / (s)	31.91 / (11.75)	12.11 / (11.08)

suffering. Table 6 gives some idea of the frequency and kind of treatments patients received during FU.

Whereas 95% of the patients had seen their GP or psychiatrist more or less regularly before treatment, only 47% had done so during follow-up, and with a lower frequency. Ratings in the second half of the table include double and triple ratings of single patients! When the low and the higher frequency visits to GP, psychiatrist and psychotherapist are taken together, treatment has reduced visits to GPs by some 75% and visits to psychiatrists and psychotherapists by some 50%. Psychotropic medication (mainly tranquilizers) was taken by 80% of the patients before exposure, but only by 25% at follow-up. This reduction in medication is not only important with regard to cost-effectiveness of treatment, but also with regard to health risks due to pharmacological treatment of

Table 6. Frequency of therapist contacts and psychotropic medication before and after exposure treatment (Average observation period 2 years)

Therapist contacts	Pre-treatment (2 year period)		During FU	
	n	%	n	%
None at all	4	(5%)	40	(53%)
≦4 per year	26	(35%)	15	(20%)
>4 per year (∅ 12 pre-treatm. ∅ 8 during FU)	45	(60%)	20	(27%)
	71	(95%)	35	(47%)
Σ	75	(100%)	75	(100%)
Kind of therapists/treatment	1–4 times		>4 times	
	Pre-treatment	Follow-up	Pre-treatment	Follow-up
General practitioner	12	6	32	5
Psychiatrist	21	12	31	15
Psychotherapist	9	3	18	11
Psychiatric hospital	5 (2 years bef. tr.) 7 (>2 years bef. tr.)	2	–	–
	Pre-treatment		During FU	
Psychotropic medication	61	(79%)	19	(25%)

agoraphobia. Agoraphobics run a strong risk to develop secondary drug dependency (tranquilizers and alcohol; cf. Wittchen, in this volume). Recently, they also seem to run a strong risk of long-term antidepressant medication, as treatment of agoraphobia with imipramin is said to be the "typical clinical practice" in the United States (Mavissakalian et al. 1983).

The question arises to what extent the treatments and medication during follow-up were able to alleviate the suffering of those patients (some 30%) who did not benefit from exposure treatment (details in 3.3.4.).

Patients' attribution of change:
Of the 59 patients who had reported improvement on a subjective improvement scale, 54 attributed this either to exposure treatment alone (20 patients) or to the combination of exposure and helpful life-events (34 patients).

Regarding exposure treatment itself, the most frequently rated positive experiences were: continuous confrontation with the real feared situation; experience of own coping skills with anxiety; and acceptance of responsibility for own actions.

How often, on the other hand, is exposure in-vivo remembered as a painful or harmful experience? 53 (70%) of the total sample (including the losers) did not report any such experiences at all. The remaining 22 (30%) mentioned the following complaints: unpleasant distress during exposure (6 patients); acute relationship problems immediately after treatment (6 patients; cf. Hand and Lamontagne 1976); brief intermittent new phobias (3 patients). The other seven patients mentioned specific individual complaints.

These complaints were reported by twelve (23%) of the 51 gainers, and ten (41%) of the losers in treatment, i.e. they are to some extent independent of treatment outcome. 56 (74%) patients suggested changes in our treatment program. Of these, 18 came out of the 24 losers (75%) and 38 out of the 51 gainers (75%), suggestions apparently being independent of treatment outcome. Several patients made more than one of the following suggestions: 28 wanted more exposure sessions and 15 more intensive pre- and post-exposure discussions; 13 (30% of the 43 who had received group exposure) wanted the groups to be more homogeneous with regard to phobic symptomatology in order to get better tailored exposure for themselves; three wanted a closer contact to their therapist in individual or group exposure, and another three more therapist contact in HBT; four would have liked a more convincing identification of the causes of their illness; finally, four would have liked to continue group treatment as a self-help group.

In essence, five of the seven groups of suggestions for change were pleas to get more of what had been given; only two asked for qualitative changes. It appears to be in the nature of man to ask for more of what feels good – even if that may not do good.

3.1.3. Comparison of Outcome with Three Different Modes of Exposure

For the comparative assessment of the effects of the three modes of exposure we computed the individual change score (T1–T4) in percentage of the ratings before treatment (percentage change score). Results (group means and standard deviation of percentage change scores), together with those of the total group, are shown in Table 7.

Eye-ball analysis seems to indicate a superiority of group exposure and HBT compared to individual exposure, and possibly a stronger anti-depressant effect of group exposure compared to HBT.

ANOVA did not reveal significance for the difference in the depression change score between group exposure and HBT. But, in social anxiety (!), total phobia and functional somatic complaints individual exposure appears significantly less effective than the other two conditions ($p < 0.001$ to $p < 0.01$).

Surprisingly, the numerically large differences between individual exposure and the two other treatments in agoraphobia are not significant. The comparatively low number of patients who received individual exposure and the high standard deviation particularly in this treatment condition require caution for an evaluation of the individual exposure in this study. This is also shown by the "subjective" improvement ratings of the patients. Of the group exposure and HBT patients some 80% rated improvement compared to some 70% of those with individual exposure – which appears a much smaller difference than in the previously reported ratings. A much more

Table 7. Symptom development over time: Percentage change scores T1 (pre) – T4 (last FU) for total group and three modes of exposure in vivo

Symptoms	Total group (n=75)		Individual exposure (n=13)		Group exposure (n=43)		Home-based treatment (n=19)	
	x̄*	(s)	x̄	(s)	x̄	(s)	x̄	(s)
Agoraphobia	39.41	(35.24)	23.55	(34.99)	41.84	(33.72)	45.39	(37.07)
Other phobias								
Social anxiety	22.66	(59.72)	–30.51	(90.32)	29.18	(45.31)	46.01	(36.15)
Phobias – total score	30.39	(30.91)	6.97	(27.06)	36.93	(30.21)	33.34	(28.33)
Other symptoms								
Depression	39.40	(54.74)	23.31	(69.22)	51.67	(35.96)	25.03	(70.89)
Obsessions-compulsions	29.14	(34.31)	25.83	(35.67)	30.03	(30.10)	29.35	(42.05)
Functional-somatic complaints	12.46	(47.24)	–23.84	(91.52)	17.75	(25.91)	25.51	(27.22)

* Group mean of percentage change score

reliable comparison of long-term effects of individual (n = 37) compared to group (n = 50) exposure will be made in our study II (5–8 years FU). Only three of the 75 patients felt worse at follow-up than before treatment, none of those came from the HBT condition.

Finally, duration of follow-up did not affect outcome results. ANOVA for FSS-agoraphobia and Marks/Watson phobia ratings (n = 75) did not reveal significant differences between any of the follow-up groups described in 2.2.

In the following two steps of analysis we shall separate the mild agoraphobics (n = 11) from those with severe agoraphobia (n = 62). Two severe agoraphobics were omitted from these analyses, as their ratings were not complete on all occasions. The detailed analyses of gainers and losers and of the two most frequently applied modes of exposure (group exposure and HBT) will be conducted with severe agoraphobics only.

3.2. Outcome of Mild Agoraphobia

We defined agoraphobia as mild when patients did not reach the cut-off point of 18 on the FSS-agoraphobia scale at pretreatment assessment. This cut-off point was empirically derived to allow a clinically meaningful definition of "severe" agoraphobia.

Eleven of the 75 patients fell into the group of mild agoraphobia. The range of their pre-treatment ratings was from 10 to 16. Group means and standard deviation on all symptom variables are shown in Table 8.

With this cut-off point it was possible to separate patients not only with regard to agoraphobic but also with regard to additional symptomatology: compared to severe agoraphobics, mild agoraphobics showed much lower ratings in other phobias and in other neurotic symptoms. In depression and obsessions-compulsions they not even reached the "clinical" range of these scales ($\geqq 10$ and $\geqq 5$ respectively). T-tests revealed significant (for resistance, interference, social anxiety and FSS-total) improvement from pre-treatment to follow-up; changes in agoraphobia are very significant, as are those in depression, although there the whole change occurred within the non-clinical range of the scale (0–10).

3.3. Outcome of Severe Agoraphobia

All subsequent comparative analyses were done with severe agoraphobics only, as we expected a higher chance for specific effects of different treatments applied to the more severely disturbed.

We shall first compare group exposure and HBT to investigate whether different cognitive sets (with regard to panic and avoidance) in both exposure modes led to different treatment outcomes. Patients with individual exposure were excluded from this analysis, as their total group of 13 included four mild agoraphobics, leaving only nine for the following comparison.

3.3.1. Comparison of Outcome with Group Exposure and Home Based Treatment

For MANOVA comparison of both treatment conditions we had to reduce the number of patients from group exposure to 19 to equal the number of HBT patients. This was done by a random procedure; subsequent comparison of both sub-groups of group exposure patients showed no differences. Results are shown in Table 9.

Table 9 only shows the ratings for the two main symptoms, agoraphobia and depression. MANOVA revealed a highly significant time-effect for both, as for the other symptom variables (not shown in Table 9), but no group effect on any of the variables. An interaction effect was only found for depression. With these results, both treatments turn out as highly and equally effective on all variables.

Nevertheless, it seems noteworthy that group exposure induced a change score of 12.34 in depression, compared to 5.39 in the HBT conditions (mean differences pretreatment to last follow-up, Table 9). From a clinical point of view this, together with the interaction effect on depression (and in spite of a missing group effect in depression), tentatively indicates an even stronger effect of group exposure on depression. Results show clearly that both modes of ex-

Table 8. Symptom development over time: special course of mild agoraphobia (n = 11)

Symptoms	Pre-treatment (T1)		Post-treatment (T2)		6-month follow-up (T3)		Last follow-up (T4)	
	x̄	(s)	x̄	(s)	x̄	(s)	x̄	(s)
Agoraphobia	14.18	(2.14)	8.60	(4.37)	10.83	(4.02)	9.92	(5.71)
Behavioral resistance	40.30	(25.10)	76.13	(12.19)	75.33	(14.14)	69.00	(23.35)
Interference	46.50	(24.74)	32.00	(21.80)	25.00	(25.16)	23.46	(19.89)
Other phobias								
Social anxiety	5.91	(4.18)	4.70	(2.67)	5.33	(4.67)	4.15	(2.51)
Phobias – total score	37.91	(13.47)	27.80	(14.68)	30.67	(11.41)	28.39	(14.60)
Other symptoms								
Depression	9.46	(6.30)	7.80	(6.23)	6.50	(7.06)	4.50	(3.89)
Obsessions-compulsions	1.82	(1.33)	1.70	(1.25)	1.67	(1.63)	1.31	(0.63)
Functional-somatic complaints	6.00	(2.22)	5.18	(2.44)	5.33	(1.97)	5.31	(1.88)

Table 9. Symptom development over time: effects of group exposure and home based treatment

Treatments	Symptoms	Pre-treatment (T1)		Post-treatment (T2)		6-month follow-up (T3)		Last follow-up (T4)	
		x̄	(s)	x̄	(s)	x̄	(s)	x̄	(s)
Group exposure (n = 19)	Agoraphobia	25.61	(6.60)	17.00	(8.10)	17.00	(8.46)	14.50	(9.87)
	Depression	22.11	(8.24)	18.00	(10.08)	16.88	(10.65)	9.77	(9.32)
Home based treatment (n = 19)	Agoraphobia	25.16	(5.75)	18.11	(7.45)	15.33	(8.24)	14.00	(9.24)
	Depression	17.72	(7.64)	13.77	(8.20)	11.77	(9.39)	12.33	(10.20)

posure are very effective treatments both for phobias and depressions. With an initial depression rating of 22.1 (group) and 17.7 (HBT), patients in both treatment conditions were far above the normal score range, whereas at follow-up scores for both groups were almost normal.

3.3.2. Comparison of Gainers and Losers

As we have already shown, combined analyses of gainers and losers may hide important, treatment-relevant information. For our comparative analyses of gainers and losers we defined as gainers patients with an FSS-agoraphobia score < 18 at last follow-up, and as losers those with ratings ≧18. Of the 62 severe agoraphobics, 39 (63%) are gainers and 23 (37%) are losers. The mean ratings of both groups separately over all assessments, and significance of differences between groups on all variables at pre-treatment and at last follow-up are shown in Table 10.

At pre-treatment, gainers and losers differ significantly only in FSS-agoraphobia. At follow-up differences between both groups are very to highly significant in all variables, except for obsession-compulsions and functional somatic complaints.

Also for this comparison we transformed ratings into percentage change scores. Comparison of change scores of gainers and losers, together with the change score for both combined, are shown in Fig. 1.

With T-tests for independent samples, differences were highly (sss) significant for FSS-agoraphobia – total score and depression, very significant (ss) for FSS-social, anxiety and significant (s) for functional so-

Table 10. Symptom development over time: comparison of gainers (n = 39) and losers (n = 23)

Symptoms	Pre-treatment (T1)		Post-treatment (T2)		6-month follow-up (T3)		Last follow-up (T4)	
	$\bar{x}$	(s)	$\bar{x}$	(s)	$\bar{x}$	(s)	$\bar{x}$	(s)
Agoraphobia								
Agoraphobia								
Gainers	22.93	(5.84)	13.05	(5.56)	11.85	(5.68)	9.05	(5.15)
(Sig. of diff.)*	s						sss	
Losers	26.52	(6.32)	21.68	(8.24)	20.63	(7.26)	23.54	(5.38)
Behavioral resistance								
Gainers	39.59	(28.03)	71.59	(20.71)	78.29	(13.58)	78.59	(20.90)
(Sig. of diff.)	n.s.						sss	
Losers	39.70	(31.31)	52.91	(21.03)	52.47	(24.98)	51.08	(25.88)
Interference								
Gainers	70.24	(21.63)	39.05	(25.50)	27.76	(23.76)	24.08	(22.75)
(Sig. of diff.)	n.s.						sss	
Losers	69.87	(19.21)	56.18	(24.50)	47.84	(25.28)	63.00	(20.94)
Other phobias								
Social anxiety								
Gainers	9.12	(4.67)	7.03	(4.77)	7.12	(4.31)	5.26	(4.03)
(Sig. of diff.)	n.s.						ss	
Losers	10.13	(4.74)	9.45	(5.63)	8.50	(3.97)	9.50	(5.18)
Phobia total score								
Gainers	60.17	(16.52)	43.19	(18.36)	39.79	(17.48)	32.56	(16.12)
(Sig. of diff.)	n.s.						sss	
Losers	67.96	(14.21)	61.14	(16.80)	60.68	(17.67)	62.63	(13.55)
Other symptoms								
Depression								
Gainers	22.51	(9.09)	14.44	(8.31)	12.47	(8.65)	8.71	(7.76)
(Sig. of diff.)	n.s.						sss	
Losers	19.95	(7.78)	18.10	(8.01)	19.11	(9.91)	18.54	(8.54)
Obsessions-compulsions								
Gainers	3.25	(1.65)	2.45	(1.57)	2.24	(1.60)	1.94	(1.46)
(Sig. of diff.)	n.s.						n.s.	
Losers	3.35	(1.95)	2.59	(2.06)	2.47	(1.87)	2.48	(1.78)
Functional somatic complaints								
Gainers	7.46	(1.61)	6.79	(1.67)	6.50	(1.99)	5.74	(2.13)
(Sig. of diff.)	n.s.						n.s.	
Losers	7.35	(1.64)	7.00	(2.14)	6.55	(2.04)	6.83	(2.17)

* Sig. of diff. ≙ t-test comparisons for independent samples: level of significances for T1 and T4

matic complaints; only for obsessions-compulsions were they non-significant. The gainers on most variables show a change score between 40% and 60% of their individual pre-treatment ratings, whereas losers show a maximum change score of 10% on only 3 variables. These extreme differences in outcome on most variables between gainers and losers do not only demonstrate their highly different responses to treatment and follow-up events, but also confirm the clinical meaningfulness of the cut-off point for FSS-agoraphobia in order to differentiate between therapeutically relevant sub-groups.

This differentiation is to a large extent possible as early as at the end of short-term treatment. Some 75% of the losers at follow-up had been losers already at the end of treatment!

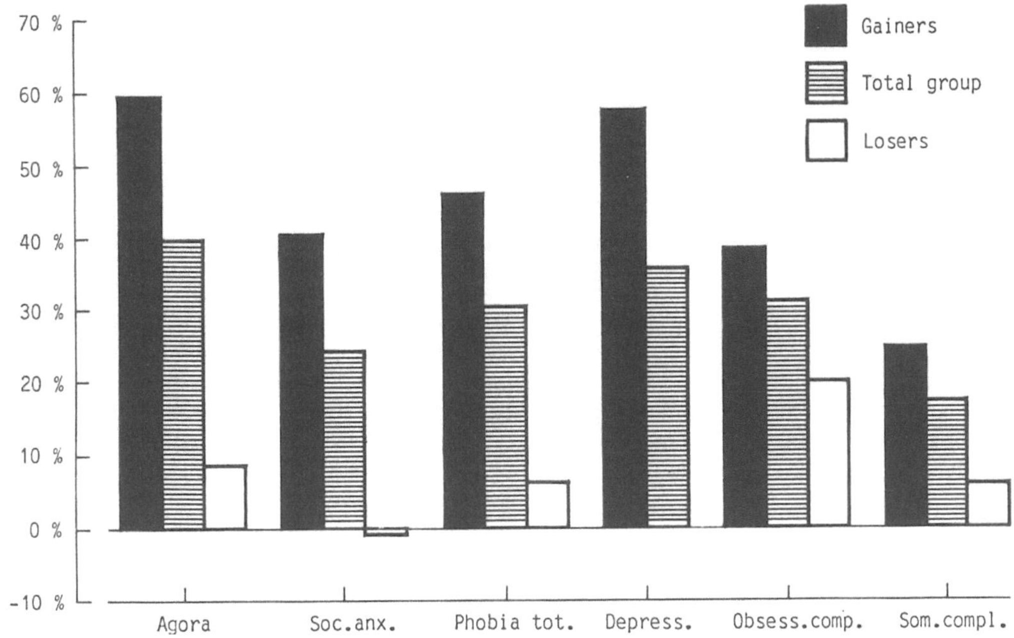

Fig. 1. Symptom development over time: percentage change-scores (T1–T4) for total group, and for gainers and losers separately

3.3.3. Level of Multisymptomatic Disturbance and Outcome in Agoraphobia

Again, we separate the gainers and losers (with regard to agoraphobia) in the described way. But now, each individual is additionally classified according to the number of additional symptoms where patients' ratings exceeded the cut-off point for the respective scale (degree of multisymptomatology): i.e. an agoraphobic will only be rated depressed in this analysis when his depression rating score reaches or exceeds the cut-off point of 23, the group mean of patients with the diagnosis of neurotic depression. Accordingly, he will only be rated obsessive-compulsive when his respective ratings reach or exceed the cut-off point of 5, which is the group mean of patients with the main diagnosis of obsessive-compulsive neurosis (details in Hand and Zaworka 1982). Cut-off points for the other two symptoms are defined in the same manner.

With this we make sure that agoraphobics who are rated as multisymptomatically disturbed have severe additional symptomatology to their agoraphobia. Results from this analysis are shown in Table 11.

Table 11. Degree of multisymptomatology and change of agoraphobia (n = 62)

Pre-treatment	Last follow-up		Σ
	Gainers	Losers	
≧ cut-off point	< cut-off point	≧ cut-off point	
Agoraphobia only	21 (70%)	9 (30%)	30
2–4 fold	18 (56%)	14 (44%)	32
symptomatology	39 (63%)	23 (37%)	62
2 fold symptomatology	5	7	12
3 fold symptomatology	10	5	15
4 fold symptomatology	3	2	5
Σ	18	14	32

Of the 30 patients who are rated monosymptomatic agoraphobics (who may still have "mild" additional symptomatology), 21 (70%) became gainers, whereas the same holds true only for 18 (56%) of the 32 with multisymptomatic disturbance. The additional, separate analysis of patients who had two-, three- or four-fold symptomatology before treatment, revealed no relationship between increasing multisymptomatology and outcome. With this evaluation procedure, patients with severe multisymptomatology show a rather high failure rate of 44% altogether.

In a next step we investigate the outcome, when multisymptomatic assessment of patients is applied for each of the three treatment conditions (Table 12).

With this analysis we get an overall success rate (percentage of gainers) of 55% in individual exposure, 71% in group exposure and 53% in HBT. The tendency for a superiority of group exposure is mainly due to the particularly high effect of group exposure in patients with severe monosymptomatic agoraphobia: of 14 patients, only one was a loser. The other differences between groups as shown in Table 12 cannot be interpreted. If these results can be confirmed, multisymptomatic assessments of individual agoraphobics (Hand and Zaworka 1982) may become a helpful screening procedure to find the most appropriate treatment for the individual patient.

3.3.4. Changes During Follow-Up

To what extent does additional symptom reduction during follow-up occur in agoraphobic patients after exposure in-vivo?

In the study by Hand et al. (1974), patients from the groups with high cohesion seem to gain further improvement during follow-up. Small numbers and short follow-ups made this a weak result, which could not be replicated, e.g. by the Oxford group. In their replication of the Hand et al. study (Teasdale et al. 1977), the lack of additional follow-up effects was the only discrepancy in outcome with the Maudsley study. In this study, with much larger samples and follow-up intervals, we could already show that except for agoraphobia in all other symptom variables there were significant to very significant follow-up effects for gainers and losers combined (Table 4). We could also show (Table 10) that on almost all variables gainers show further numerical improvement from post-treatment to last FU. A more detailed analysis of FU effects on all symptom variables for the 62 severe agoraphobics is shown in Table 13.

Reanalysis of the total sample reveals follow-up effects very similar to those shown in Table 4 for the total sample of 75 patients, including the mild agoraphobics. For the gainers we now find significant to very significant follow-up effects also in the three dimensions of agoraphobia – an effect which was spurred by the development of the losers in the joint analysis. The significance of follow-up improvement in depression increases further in the separate analysis for the gainers.

These clear-cut results of very significant treatment as well as follow-up improvement on all symptom variables for gainers as opposed to losers give much clearer hints about treatment effects than the usual combined analysis of gainers and losers.

A closer look at the development of the losers reveals that of the 23 losers, 19 had received some kind of treatment during fol-

Table 12. Degree of multisymptomatology and change of agoraphobia after three different modes of exposure in-vivo

Pre-treatment	Last FU						Σ
Symptomatology ≧ cut-off point	Ind. exposure n=9		Group exposure n=34		Home Based Treatment n=19		
	Gainers	Losers	Gainers	Losers	Gainers	Losers	
Agoraphobia only	1	2	13	1	7	6	30 (48%)
2–4 fold symptomatology	4	2	11	9	3	3	32 (52%)
Σ	5 (55%)	4 (45%)	24 (71%)	10 (29%)	10 (53%)	9 (47%)	62 (100%)

Table 13. Symptom development over time: Follow-up effects (T2–T4) for total sample, and for gainers and losers seperately

Symptoms	Total sample (n=62)			Gainers (n=39)			Losers (n=23)		
	T*	p	sig.	T*	p	sig.	T*	p	sig.
Agoraphobia									
Agoraphobia	1.72	0.090	n.s.	3.31	0.002	ss	−1.14	0.266	n.s.
Behavioral resistance	−1.42	0.161	n.s.	−2.72	0.010	s	1.04	0.310	n.s.
Interference	1.74	0.087	n.s.	2.95	0.006	ss	−0.99	0.335	n.s.
Other phobias									
Social anxiety	1.81	0.075	n.s.	3.01	0.005	ss	−0.40	0.693	n.s.
Phobias – total score	2.34	0.023	s	3.71	0.001	ss	−0.37	0.711	n.s.
Other symptoms									
Depression	2.49	0.016	s	4.05	0.000	sss	−0.59	0.558	n.s.
Obsessions-compulsions	2.40	0.021	s	2.92	0.007	ss	0.0	1.00	n.s.
Functional-somatic complaints	3.14	0.003	ss	3.69	0.001	ss	0.41	0.685	n.s.

* T-tests for dependent samples

low-up (not behavior therapy), one was on a waiting list for additional behavior therapy – and three asked for more behavior therapy at follow-up. Also a certain proportion of the gainers received further treatments during follow-up.

Of 19 patients with psychotropic medication at follow-up, twelve were losers (i.e. 51% of the losers) and seven were gainers (17% of the gainers). None of the mild agoraphobics received medication at follow-up.

Twenty three patients saw their therapists (GPs, psychiatrists or psychotherapists) on a more regular basis during follow-up. Fifteen of these were losers (65% of the losers), seven were gainers (18% of the gainers), and one was a mild agoraphobic.

Treatments during follow-up altogether emphasize the differences between gainers and losers, revealed by their symptom ratings.

Losers in 75% are detectable already at the end of short-term exposure. They receive much more additional treatment during follow-up than gainers and yet, whereas gainers continue to gain in follow-up, losers hardly ever do so.

4. Summary and Discussion

This study reveals a variety of results not found, or not looked for, in previous follow-up studies with agoraphobics. This may to some extent be due to the way treatments were conducted, but it is probably much more the consequence of some new ways of data analysis. Data analyses start with an initial, "classical" analysis of the total patient sample, including a comparison and three modes of exposure (individual, group and home-based). This is followed by an analysis with the subsample of "mild" agoraphobics (11, or 15% of the total sample). The most informative analyses are then conducted with the severely disturbed patients. Comparison of treatment conditions in this sample, because of the small number of patients with individual exposure, is restricted to group exposure and home-based treatment in most analyses. Severe agoraphobics are then split into gainers and losers, according to their phobia ratings at last follow-up. Possible reasons for the differences in their rating at follow-up, in spite of their homogeneity at pre-treatment, are carefully analysed. In this context, separate analyses of treatment and follow-up effects are of special interest, as apart from some first tentative results in the Hand et al. study (1974), so far additional follow-up effects could not be detected after exposure treatment of agoraphobics.

The experimental section of this study is introduced by a rather detailed description of the "exposure-response management" model of group exposure in-vivo (Hand et al. 1974), as the response-management part of it seems to have been largely neglected in subsequent studies. Differences for the coping strategy in home-based treatment (Mathews et al. 1977) are outlined. These treatment descriptions are hoped to contribute to a conceptual plausibility of some major outcomes of the study.

Overall outcomes:
Analyses with the data from the whole sample confirm previous follow-up studies with agoraphobics regarding highly significant phobia reduction and very positive changes in private and professional life, as well as in illness behavior. Additionally, highly significant effects of treatment are found in multisymptomatology, including depression, social anxiety, obsessions-compulsions and functional somatic complaints. Also, on all variables except the directly treated agoraphobia, there is further significant improvement during follow-up. The intense changes in agoraphobic behavior right after treatment may have had lasting effects on life style, which in turn additionally may have reduced other symptomatology. Results on assessor-administered multiple scales confirm the outcome with patient's self-ratings. At follow-up, only 30% of the total sample still suffer from considerable to severe symptomalogy. For the other 70%, the marked reduction in phobic anxiety is accompanied by marked increase in psychological well-being, occupational and leisure activities. Compared to pre-treatment, visits to GPs have been reduced by 75%, those to psychiatrists and psychotherapists by 50%. Psychotropic medication had been taken by 80% before treatment, while only 25% were still taking it at follow-up. Thus, treatment also reduced health risks secondary to agoraphobia, like drug dependency (tranquilizers or alcohol) and the risks of long-term anti-depressant medication.

Some 90% of the improved patients attributed improvement to behavior therapy alone or in combination with other life events. They also said they would go back to behavior therapy if again in need of help. Yet quite a large proportion of the patients (gainers and losers) made a variety of suggestions to improve treatment: in most cases patients would have liked more of what they had got, rather than change anything. It appears to be in the nature of man to ask for more of what feels good – even if that may not do good.

Group statistical analyses with this sample revealed the high efficacy of both group exposure and home-based treatment with no specific superior effect of either on any of the variables.

Duration of follow-up did not affect outcome.

Thus, in the first overall analysis it appears that short-term exposure of whatever mode induces such intense changes in phobic and everyday behavior that more than two thirds of treatment participants after the initiation of change by treatment continued to change their lives during follow-up.

Results with mild agoraphobics:
Mild agoraphobics in this study are those that before treatment scored lower than our clinical cut-off point of 18 on the FSS-agoraphobia scale. With this cut-off point, we not only separated patients with regard to agoraphobia, but also with regard to the level of additional multisymptomatology from the severe agoraphobics (cf. Table 8 versus Table 10). Mild agoraphobics are in the large majority monosymptomatically disturbed: in depression, obsession-compulsions and functional somatic complaints their ratings are well within the normal range of the respective scales; in social anxiety and FSS-total phobia score they are far below our clinical cut-off points for severe symptomatology.

Mild agoraphobics apparently start treatment with a phobia level (14, 18) that almost equals that of the total sample at last follow-up (13, 76) – and yet, they gain considerably and significantly in phobia as well as in "normal" depression.

Results with severe agoraphobics:
The first analysis with the sample of 62 patients consists of a comparison of treatment and follow-up effects of patients after *group exposure* or *home-based treatment.* MANOVA revealed highly significant effects on all variables, but no group effect. Both treatments show particularly strong effects on phobic anxiety, group exposure additionally on depression (change score 11,1 compared to 5,4 in HBT). This result, and the only significant MANOVA interaction effect occurring in depression, tentatively support the assumption of a specifically powerful group exposure effect on depression – in spite of the missing group effect. From the different anxiety-depression management concepts in both treatment modes, these differences in outcome seem to make sense. Group exposure tries to induce high emotional arousal and uses almost identical coping strategies for panic and depression. As already mentioned in the original study, high group cohesion may be the optimal motivational setting for proper application of this treatment mode. There is also further evidence, that group exposure might have some specific advantages over home-based treatment: in monosymptomatic severe agoraphobics (Table 11), of the 14 who had received group exposure, 13 (93%) turned out gainers at follow-up, whereas the same holds true for only 7 (54%) of the 13 who had received home-based treatment. Again, the lack of an active coping strategy for high emotional arousal (here: anxiety-panic) in HBT may explain these differences in outcome. Unfortunately, in this study we did not apply rating scales to properly assess occurrence of panic in and outside phobic situations.

In severe multisymptomatic agoraphobics we did not find differences in outcome between treatments, all being successful in somewhat more than 50% of the patients. It may not be the same 50% of the patients that profit from each of the treatment conditions, but the so far small numbers did not allow more detailed analyses. Taking all results together, some tentative first suggestions for treatment settings that are equipped to provide both modes of exposure seem justified: patients with 1. severe, monosymptomatic agoraphobia and (or) 2. high, phobia-related depression may preferably be treated by group exposure in-vivo.

The separate analysis of *gainers* (n = 39; 63%) and *losers* (n = 23, 37%) among the severe agoraphobics – independent of treatment conditions – reveals the most useful information from the study. Gainers were those patients who, with a pre-treatment rating of $\geqq 18$ in FSS-agoraphobia, scored < 18 at last follow-up. Theoretically, with this cut-off point gainers could still be mild agoraphobics in our definition. Pre-treatment, both groups differed significantly only in the agoraphobia ratings (initially higher in losers), whereas at follow-up differences in all symptom variables, except for obsession-compulsions and functional somatic complaints, were highly significant (Table 10). Gainers on most variables had a change score of 40–60% of their individual pre-treatment ratings, whereas losers showed a maximum change score of 10% and this only in three variables. Our cut-off point thus has proved a very useful tool to differentiate between responders and non-responders to treatment, even on a multi-symptomatic level.

Results also show that those who had responded at last follow-up, had done so during treatment as well as additionally during follow-up (Table 13). Gainers show significant additional follow-up effects on all variables of phobic and additional symptomatology, whereas losers show no such effects at all. In gainers for instance, continuing change during follow-up is the reason why they did not remain mild agoraphobics: they scored 13.05 at the end of treatment (whereas mild agoraphobics had scored 14 before treatment), but 9.05 at last follow-up, thus finishing with an almost identical rating to the last follow-up of mild agoraphobics (9.92).

Additional treatments during follow-up had occurred far more often in losers than in gainers: 51% of the losers compared to 17% of the gainers took psychotropic medication at follow-up (none of the mild agoraphobics); 65% of the losers and 18% of the gainers had seen their therapists (GPs, psychiatrists or psychotherapists) on a more regular basis during follow-up. Yet, losers had remained losers, even when treated with alternative psychotherapy.

Why did losers become losers and stay losers? With the detailed analysis of losers still under way, here we can only give some tentative suggestions. During treatment and the first six months of follow-up all variables except for depression show at least a numerical tendency for symptom reduction (Table 10). Only depression ratings remain highly stable over this period of time as well as during subsequent follow-up. This happened in spite of the fact that the initial depression ratings of losers (19, 95) and gainers (22, 51) were very similar. Why then did depression of the losers respond so extremely differently to depression of the gainers? Two hypothetical explanations need further investigation: 1. Was the initial behavioral analysis wrong with regard to the symptom and problem hierarchy of the losers? Was the cause of multisymptomatology one major, "underlying" problem or conflict that we did not detect more properly? But why then did patients not respond to alternative treatments in follow-up? 2. Did losers suffer from some basic biological depression-anxiety (panic) disturbance? Interestingly, losers had a significantly higher rating of phobic anxiety than gainers prior to treatment – in contrast to their numerically lower depression ratings.

In both cases (1. and 2.), chronic, non-respondent depression would then be seen as due to an underlying cause other than agoraphobia, this also being the cause for relapses in the responding variables after six-month follow-up.

Another sub-sample of the losers, those 25% who came from the post-treatment gainers, needs further investigation, possibly in the same directions.

It needs to be added again that, from the interviews and the experience of patients in treatment, the occurrence of panic attacks does not seem to correlate with persistent depression in treatment and during follow-up. The existence of a non-responding depression may have to be detected from other variables.

The separate analysis of gainers and losers convincingly demonstrates how the "classical" total sample group statistics can hide important, and may even give wrong information. In our initial, total sample analysis, patients finished treatment with a mean agoraphobia score of almost 14, which could have led to the wrong assumption that even a long time after exposure patients, in spite of their improvement, are still mild, though definite agoraphobics in need of treatment. Only the detailed subanalyses described reveal that for the clear majority exposure is highly effective during treatment as well as during follow-up and on a multisymptomatic level, or it is not effective at all, losers apparently also hardly responding to alternative treatments.

Prognostic variables for the course of agoraphobia in exposure treatment and during follow-up:

1. Responsiveness of phobia *and* depression during short-term exposure is a strong predictor of positive long-term outcome for some two thirds of the patients. If both variables respond, the level of depression before treatment does not affect outcome negatively. In fact, both modes of exposure are then powerful "anti-phobic" as well as "anti-depressant" interventions.

Occurrence of panic attacks during group exposure in-vivo appears to be a good predictor for positive short-term outcome, as we found in a previous study.

On the other hand, non-responders in depression during phobia treatment are likely to remain non-responders in depression during follow-up – thus indicating the high risk of relapse after six month follow-up in all variables that may have responded favorably to treatment. Early separation of gainers and losers with a single-case oriented methodology like that one described by Hand and Zaworka (1982) seems warranted.

2. Selection of the proper mode of exposure for the individual patient may be important

in some sub-samples of agoraphobics, in spite of the almost equal, highly significant multisymptomatic effects of both HBT and group exposure. Patients with severe monosymptomatic agoraphobia, and possibly also those with higher phobia-related depression, seem to profit better from group exposure. The same would go for those who want to improve as fast as possible and to travel as far as possible. On the other hand, those who want time, who want to avoid emotional arousal, who want to exercise according to their own speed, who have been identified as severely multisymptomatic patients, and finally those who cannot find a trained exposure therapist, may very well turn to HBT.

The following questions arise from this study:

1. Why does, in some 30% of severe agoraphobics, depression not respond to phobia-treatment, while in the other 70% exposure treatment is a very effective anti-depressant intervention? Is the non-responding depression a symptom of a psychological problem or conflict constellation, or is it of biological origin? Why did losers in this study neither respond to alternative treatments nor to medications?
2. Why do severely multisymptomatic agoraphobics respond only in 50% favorably to treatment, compared to 93% of the severely monosymptomatic agoraphobics (in group exposure)? What relationship is there between level of phobic anxiety on one side and level of depression on the other side and the level of multisymptomatology? To a certain extent, higher levels of phobic anxiety correlate with higher degrees of multisymptomatology – mild agoraphobics have virtually no other symptoms of clinical relevance, whereas 50% of severe agoraphobics have stilt other severe symptoms.

How can we identify those 50% of the severely multisymptomatic patients who do not respond to exposure, before the intervention is given?
3. Can our hypothesis about some specific effects of group exposure be verified in an additional controlled trial with HBT and group exposure? Such a study should also investigate the exact occurrence of panic attacks (according to DSM-III) to investigate whether there is really the assumed specific "anti-panic" and "anti-depression" effect of the *exposure response-management* concept already inherent in the group exposure in-vivo model by Hand et al. (1974). This comprises "exposure to the avoided trigger situation and (or) to the feared own set of responses" – the latter being cognitive, emotional (anxiety, depression or other) or physiological.

In spite of all the questions yet to be answered, from this study there is already one reassuring answer: for 70% of agoraphobics group exposure or HBT are highly effective and sufficient treatments. In the majority, long-term gainers and losers can be identified already at the end of treatment. Doubts that have come up from some studies oriented at a biological panic model cannot at all be confirmed by this large-scale and long-term study.

5. References

Agras WS, Berkowitz R (1980) Clinical research in behavior therapy: Halfaway there? Behavior Therapy 9:472–487

Bandura A (1978) Self-efficacy: Toward a unifying theory of behavioral change. In: Francks CM, Wilson GT (eds) Annual Review of Behavior Therapy: Theory and Practice (Vol. 6) Brunner & Mazel, New York

Barlow DH, Wolfe BE (1981) Behavioral approaches to anxiety disorders: A report on the NIMH-SUNY, Albany research conference. J Cons Clin Psychol 49:448–454

Chambless DL, Golstein AJ (1981) Clinical treatment of agoraphobia. In: Chambless DL, Goldstein AJ (eds) Phobia: Psychological and pharmacological treatment. Guilford, New York

Cohen SD, Monteiro W, Marks IM (1984) Two-year follow-up of agoraphobics after exposure and imipramine. Br J Psychiatry 144:276–287

Emmelkamp PMG, Kuipers AC (1979) Agoraphobia: A follow-up study four years after treatment. Br J Psychiatry 134:352–355

Fahrenberg J (1975) Die Freiburger Beschwerdeliste, FBL. Zeitschrift für klinische Psychologie 4:79–100

Fahrenberg J, Selg H, Hampel R (1973) Das Freiburger Persönlichkeitsinventar, FPI. Handanweisung. Hogrefe, Göttingen

Fahrenberg J, Selg H, Hampel R (1984) Das Freiburger Persönlichkeitsinventar, FPI. Handanweisung der revidierten Fassung FPI-R und der teilweise geänderten Fassung FPI-A. Hogrefe, Göttingen

Foa FB, Emmelkamp PMG (eds) (1983) Failures in behavior therapy. Wiley, New York

Hafner RJ, Marks IM (1976) Exposure in vivo of agoraphobics: contributions of diazepam, group exposure and anxiety evocation. Psychol Med 6:71–88

Hallam RS, Hafner RJ (1978) Fears of phobic patients. Factor analyses of self-report data. Beh Res Ther 16:1–6

Hand I (1984) Verhaltenstherapie und Psychopharmaka bei Phobien? Welche Konsequenzen hat die „Entdeckung" der Panic Disorder wirklich für die verhaltenstherapeutische Praxis und Forschung? In: Götze P (ed) Leitsymptom Angst. Springer, Berlin

Hand I (1986) Verhaltenstherapie und kognitive Therapie in der Psychiatrie. In: Kisker KP, Lanter H, Meyer J-E, Müller C, Strömgen E (eds) Psychiatrie der Gegenwart, Band 1, 3. Auflage. Springer, Berlin Heidelberg New York

Hand I, Lamontagne Y (1976) The exacerbation of interpersonal problems after rapid phobia-removal. Psychotherapy: Theory, Research and Practice 13:405–411

Hand I, Lamontagne Y, Marks IM (1974) Group exposure (flooding) in vivo for agoraphobics. Br J Psychiatry 124:588–602

Hand I, Schröder G (1980) Die vago-vasale Ohnmacht bei der Blut-Verletzungs-Katastrophen (BVK)-Phobie und ihre verhaltenstherapeutische Behandlung. Therapiewoche 30:923–932

Klein D (1981) Anxiety reconceptualized. In: Klein D, Rabkin J (eds) Anxiety: New Research and changing concept. Raven Press, New York

Lambert MJ, Bergin AE (1978) The evaluation of therapeutic outcome. In: Garfield SC, Bergin AE (eds) Handbook of psychotherapy and behavior change: An empirical analysis. Wiley, New York

Mahoney M (1983) Cognition, consciousness and processes of personal change. In: Craig K, McMahon R (eds) Advances in clinical behavior therapy. Brunner & Mazel, New York

Marks IM (1970) The classification of phobic disorders. Br J Psychiatry 116:337–380

Marks IM (1971) Phobic disorders four years after treatment: A prospective follow-up. Br J Psychiatry 118:683–688

Marks IM (1975) Behavioral treatment of phobic and obsessive-compulsive disorders: a critical appraisal. In: Hersen M, Eisler R, Miller P (eds) Progress in behavior modification. Academic Press, New York

Marks IM (1983) Panic attacks in phobia: treatment studies. Arch Gen Psychiatry 40:1151

Mathews AM, Teasdale J, Munby M, Johnston D, Shaw P (1977) A home based treatment program for agoraphobia. Behavior Therapy 8:915–924

Mathews A, Gelder M, Johnston D (1981) Agoraphobia. Nature and treatment. Guilford Press, New York

Mavissakalian M, Michelson L, Dealy S (1983) Pharmacological treatment of agoraphobia: Imipramine versus Imipramine with programmed practice. Br J Psychiatry 143:348–355

McPherson FM, Brougham L, McLaren S (1980) Maintainance of improvement in agoraphobic patients treated by behavioral methods – a four year follow-up. Behav Res Ther 8:150–152

Munby M, Johnston DW (1980) Agoraphobia: The long-term follow-up of behavioral treatment. Brit J Psychiatry 137:418–427

Nie NH, Hull CM, Jenkins K, Bent DH (1980) SPSS – Statistical Package for the Social Sciences. McGraw Hill, New York

Priebe S (1980) Die Bedeutung von Kohäsion und Angstfluktuation bei Kurzzeitübungs-Gruppen von Agoraphobikern. Unveröffentlichte Dissertation. Universität Hamburg

Sheehan D, Ballenger J, Jacobsen G (1980) Treatment of endogenous anxiety with phobic hysterical and hypochondrical symptoms. Arch Gen Psychiatry 37:51–59

Shipley R, Boudewyns P (1980) Flooding and implosive therapy: Are they harmful? Behavior Therapy 11:503–508

Strian F (1983) Angst. Grundlagen und Klinik. Springer, Berlin

Tearnan BH, Telch MJ (1984) Phobic disorders. In: Adams HE, Sutker PB (eds) Comprehensive handbook of psychopathology. Plenum Press, New York London

Teasdale JD, Walsh PA, Lancashire M, Mathews AM (1977) Group exposure for agoraphobics: A replication study. Brit J Psychiatry 130:186–193

Thorpe G, Burns L (1983) The Agoraphobic syndrome. Wiley, New York Chichester

Thorpe GL, Burns LE, Smith PJ, Blier MJ (1984) Agoraphobia: Research developments and clinical implications. In: Franks CM (ed) New developments in behavior therapy from research to clinical application. The Haworth Press, New York

Watson JP, Marks IM (1971) Relevant and irrelevant fear in flooding – a crossover study of phobic patients. Behavior Therapy 2:275–293

Zaworka W, Hand I, Jauernig G, Lünenschloß K (1983) Das Hamburger Zwangsinventar (HZI) Manual and Fragebogen. Beltz, Weinheim

Zerssen von DV, Koeller D-M (1976) Klinische Selbstbeurteilungsskalen (KSb-S) aus dem Münchener psychiatrischen Informationssystem. Beltz, Weinheim

Zitrin C, Klein D, Woerner M (1980) Treatment of agoraphobia with group exposure in vivo and imipramine. Arch Gen Psychiatry 37:63–72

Subject Index

MIX
Papier aus verantwortungsvollen Quellen
Paper from responsible sources
FSC® C105338

If you have any concerns about our products,
you can contact us on
ProductSafety@springernature.com

In case Publisher is established outside the EU,
the EU authorized representative is:
Springer Nature Customer Service Center GmbH
Europaplatz 3, 69115 Heidelberg, Germany

Printed by Libri Plureos GmbH
in Hamburg, Germany